How to make

Infusions and Decoctions

Book One of the Herbal Preparations Series

By Starr Morgayne

How to make Infusions and Decoctions by Starr Morgayne

How to make

Infusions and Decoctions

Book One of the Herbal Preparations Series

Written by Starr Morgayne

Cover Design by Starr Morgayne

Published by

Dark Moon Press

P.O. Box 11496

Fort Wayne, Indiana 46858-1496

www.DarkMoonPress.com

DarkMoon@DarkMoonPress.com

ISBN-13: 978-1493503650

Health & Fitness/Herbal Medicine

How to make Infusions and Decoctions by Starr Morgayne

Other Books by Starr Morgayne

Bewitching Beauty; Bringing out your inner Goddess, naturally

How to Make Salves; Book Two in the Herbal Preparations Series

How to Make Tinctures and Glycerites; Book Three in the Herbal Preparations Series

How to Make Lotions and Creams; Book Four in the Herbal Preparations Series

How to make Infusions and Decoctions by Starr Morgayne

Disclaimer

The information contained within this book is presented solely for general informational purposes only. Nothing contained in this book is intended to constitute, nor should it be considered, medical advice. It should not serve as a substitute for the advice of a physician or other qualified health care provider. I make no assurances of the information being suited to your medical needs and, to the maximum extent allowed by law, disclaim any and all warranties and liabilities related to your use of any of the information and/or recipes obtained from within these pages. Please make sure to keep in mind any allergies and/or dietary concerns when working with plants and other ingredients.

The information provided in this book should not be considered complete, nor should it be relied on to suggest a course of treatment for a particular individual, nor is it intended to refer you to a particular medical professional or health care provider. It should not be used as a substitute for a visit to, consultation with or the advice of a physician or other qualified health care provider.

Information obtained from within this book is not exhaustive and does not cover all diseases, ailments or physical conditions or their treatment. Should you have any health care related questions, call or see your physician or other qualified health care provider promptly. You should never disregard medical advice or delay in seeking it because of something you have read in this book.

How to make Infusions and Decoctions by Starr Morgayne

Table of Contents

Introduction

Taking care of people and helping them heal has always interested me. I think that might stem from my grandmother being a nurse and my mother wanting to follow in those footsteps. I, however, went in a slightly different direction.

I was always curious about different plant life. My mother had a large garden where she grew many vegetables and I enjoyed helping her in the garden and smelling the vegetables as they grew.

My mother is very much a plant lover and so we had many houseplants all around. Because of this, one of my science fair projects in Junior High was studying the growth of plants and how outside stimuli affected them. One of the things that I found out is that talking to and playing music for them helped them grow immensely and to this day when I water my little lovelies I tell them how proud of them I am and how beautiful they're looking.

I very much enjoyed picking things from the garden and making meals out of it. The produce that I would walk along the aisles grazing upon always tasted so much better than the everyday grocery store fare.

My love of making things, as well as my love of herbs and other plants, grew as I got older. In my late teens I became interested in my Native American heritage. I began going to powwows and creating Native American style jewelry. This got me even more interested in how my ancestors lived. I began studying what foods they ate and how they healed themselves through food and natural medicines. This got me started with making teas, bath bags, salves, etc.

Thanks to random chance I met up with a woman who would change my life. Through her teachings I learned so much more. I slept in a tipi on her property many times. I picked St. John's Wort in her meadow, helped build an arch for the gourds in her garden, scraped a deer hide to get it ready for tanning, fed chickens, watched the sun rise and the rabbits hop across the field as the deer grazed, suffered through many a sweat lodge ceremony and loved every minute of it.

2

Since that time I have continued on with my study of herbs, alternative medicine, naturopathy (healing through food) and Native cultures.

My days now are spent caring for my zoo of animals, my family and creating even more salves, lotions, potions, brews, teas and anything else I can think of.

I wanted to write this book so that I can share with you, the reader, my love of everything natural as well as the knowledge I have gained throughout my time here.

Many of the things that we need to sustain ourselves, keep ourselves healthy and make ourselves beautiful is right in our own backyards, sometimes literally.

This is, in my opinion, a healthier and more harmonious way of going about things. It is also more in accordance with our own bodies and helps them work in a more natural manner.

The information contained in this book has come from many different sources too numerous to name. In all of these years I have grown, researched and learned more than I could imagine. I hope that I can encourage you to do the same.

If you have any questions about ingredients or definitions of terms used within these pages I have included a glossary of terms as well as an ingredient list at the end of this book. Many of your questions may be answered there.

If you cannot find the answer to your questions within these pages, I encourage you to contact me through my publisher, Dark Moon Press (DarkMoon@DarkMoonPress.com), Facebook (https://www.facebook.com/StarrMorgayne), or research the information on your own.

Infusions

What is an infusion? The word "infusion" comes from the root "infuse". According to Merriam-Webster, infuse means "to cause to be permeated with something (as a principle or quality) that alters usually for the better <*infuse* the team with confidence".

In the case of this book, an infusion is what you get when you use a liquid to pull the needed constituents of an herb out of the plant matter and into the liquid.

To protect your infusions when they are finished you are going to want to keep them away from heat and light. There are many places where you can get amber or cobalt blue colored bottles to store your infusions in.

Always make sure to do your research when making any sort of herbal preparation. Make sure that the herb(s) you are using are not poisonous or that whomever may be using the preparation doesn't have any allergies to the herbs that you have incorporated into it.

Using Fresh Plants

If you are using fresh plants make sure you know exactly what plant you are using and what that plant does as well as what parts of the plant are best to use for what you are trying to accomplish. If you use the wrong plant because it looks like another, or you're not sure what it is, the effects can be harmful and even sometimes fatal. If you're using the wrong part of the plant, even if you are using the correct plant, you may not get the results that you're looking for in the preparation that you are creating. You may need the bark instead of the leaves or you might need the root instead of the petals of the flower. Always make sure you've done your homework before putting anything together.

Because fresh plant material still has moisture in it there is a possibility that with certain recipes (such as infused oils) you may get some mold growth. In order to avoid this make sure to cover all of the plant material with oil and you can also add a natural preservative such as Vitamin E or Grapefruit Seed Extract while you are storing your infusion.

Using Dried Plants

If you are using dried plant material you want to make sure that it has maintained its color and scent. Crush or rub a little in your hands and smell it to make sure, if you need to. If you aren't able to crush and smell the herbs take a look at their color. If the herbs are dull and

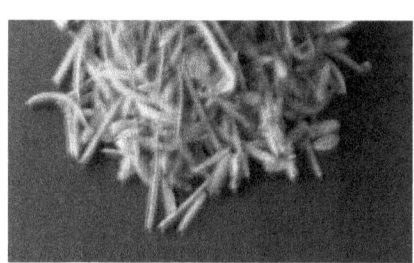 brown looking they have lost their potency. If the herb is meant to be brown, such as Cinnamon or Cloves, look at the intensity of the color. Herbs that maintain a bright color will usually have maintained their potency as well. Another thing to remember, when using dried herbs, is that you'll usually want to replace them every 6 months or so. I have been able to keep herbs for longer than that but you always need to check the color and scent. Often times I'll use older herbs for crafts where the potency is not such a big issue.

If you're using a recipe that calls for a certain amount of fresh herbs you'll need less of the dried herbs. The ratio most commonly used is usually 2 to 1 (or ½ the

amount of dried herb as compared to fresh). If your recipe calls for two tablespoons of fresh herb then you should be able to use one tablespoon of dried herb and vice versa.

Some plants work just as well in dried form as they do fresh but some do not. In some cases you will need the vital oils from the fresh plant in order to accomplish the goal of whatever you are creating.

Always make sure to store your herbs away from light and heat in order to keep them fresher longer. Storing them in a cabinet can help with this. My family often jokes that I need my own "herb cabinet" the size of a small bedroom.

Powdered herbs will lose the efficacy the quickest. Once the herbs are ground into a powder their essential oils will dissipate rapidly. I don't usually use powdered herbs to make infusions. If I do need to use the powdered form of an herb I will usually either dry it myself or purchase it in dried form then grind it into a powder with my coffee grinder.

Some herbs have properties that are better extracted in water and some properties that are better extracted through oil. Common Plantain is one example. You can make a water infusion and an oil infusion, separately of course, to extract both types of properties from the plant and then combine them, along with an emulsifying agent, into a healing cream.

There are many ways to make an herbal infusion and we will discuss them in this chapter. We will also discuss the myriad of ways in which you can use an herbal infusion.

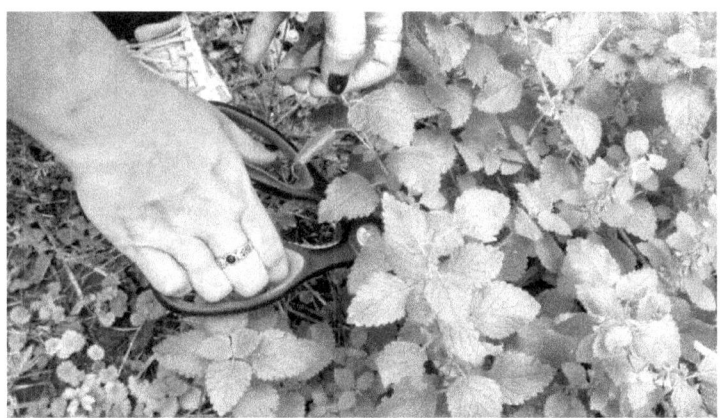

Collecting Lemon Balm from my yard to make an infusion.

At the end of this book you will find recipes in which to use your infusions. I hope you enjoy them and that it inspires you to come up with some recipes of your own.

Different types of Infusions

Infusions can be made using water, oil, Honey, vinegar, alcohol and/or glycerine. Infusions made using alcohol or glycerine are known as Tinctures (alcohol or vinegar) and Glycerites (glycerine). Those will be discussed in Book Three of this series.

Infusions are best to use for the more fragile parts of the plants such as petals, whole flowers, leaves and some seeds and/or berries.

You can use one particular plant or you can use a combination of several different types of plants and/or plant material to create your infusions.

Different parts of the plant will require different steeping times so you want to make sure that you don't the two at the same time or you could end up with a very bitter tasting infusion. Just make your infusions separately and then combine them when they are both finished.

Herbs that have a better flavor are often infused with herbs that may already have a bitter or unpleasant taste. For example, sometimes Mint is added to tea recipes in order to add a more pleasant flavor.

Water Infusions

A water infusion is more commonly known as an "herbal tea". They are also known as "tisanes". There is a slight difference between a tea and a general infusion. An infusion usually contains a larger quantity of plant material and is steeped longer and therefore contains more of the nutrients that the plant material has to offer. The longer you steep your infusion the more the liquid has time to pull out the constituents of the plant material. According to several sources, a cup of Nettle tea has 5-10 mg of calcium, while a cup of Nettle infusion can contain up to 500 mg of calcium!

Water infusions can be made in many different ways but the basics of an infusion are using heat and/or time to cause the healing components of the herb to be pulled out of the plant matter into the carrier component, which, in this case, is water. Water infusions are often touted as the best way to get medicinal herbs and plants into the body.

Ways to make water infusions

There are a couple of different ways to make water infusions. Keep in mind that a water infusion will not last long on its own, usually only about 12 hours or less, so don't be tempted to make too much at once. However, you can freeze a strained and cooled infusion in an ice-cube tray and keep it in your freezer for up to three months. According to famed herbalist Susun Weed, dried herbs are best because "the minerals and other phytochemicals in nourishing herbs are made more accessible by drying".

The most common way is to make a tea by boiling the water (not a rolling boil) over a stove or fire and pouring it over the dried herbs. Allow the infusion to steep for ten to thirty minutes before straining. When the infusion is steeping you want to keep it covered so that the essential oils are not released into the air through the steam that is rising from the water. The longer the infusion steeps the stronger it will be.

Strain the plant material from the liquid using cheesecloth, a coffee filter, a French Press, or any other way you feel comfortable. If you're using cheesecloth or something similar you can wrap it up like a little bundle, twist up the top so nothing comes out and squeeze it with your hands to get as much of the oil out as possible. It is a messy process but well worth it. You want to make sure that you have been able to remove any of the particles left over from the plant material itself. You can then compost your leftover plant material and store your infusion or use it.

You can also put the plant material into tea bags which are a filter all on their own. You can buy tea bags that already contain the herbs that you are looking to use or ones that are open on one end so that you can fill them with the herb(s) of your choice and then seal them yourself. If you purchase the open ended tea bags you can fill them with your plant material and seal the end with a hot iron. When I make a lot of tea bags at once I will use the sealing strip on my food vacuum sealer to close the end of the bags. It allows me to do more than one bag at a time and does a great job of getting them sealed properly.

If you are making a medicinal beverage the general dosage recommendation is two to four cups a day.

You can also make solar infusions using water. Sun tea is one example of a solar water infusion.

To make a solar infusion you will want to gather up your herbal material and place it in a clean jar with a lid. Put a label on the jar with all of the information you will need: the name of the herb you are using, the type of infusion (water, oil, etc.), the date in which you started the infusion and the date in which the infusion should be ready to use (about two to four weeks later depending on the weather for oil infusions and a few hours for a water infusion). Fill the jar with the herb(s) leaving at least one inch of space between the top of the jar and the plant material. After you have filled your jar with the herbal material you must then fill it with water until it is just over the top of the herbs if you want a very strong infusion. For a less strong infusion, of course, you will want to use less of the plant material. Make sure that all of the plant material is covered to help avoid any growth of bacteria or fungi. Place the jar on a sunny windowsill, or any other sunny location, where it won't be bothered during steeping.

After the appropriate amount of time, you will want to remove the jar from its sunny location and strain the plant material from the liquid using cheesecloth, a coffee filter, a French Press, or any other way you feel comfortable. You want to make sure that you have been able to remove any of the particles left over from the plant material. You can then store your infusion or use it.

Water infusions can be used as beverages (teas are one example), hair rinses, facial steams, made into lotions and/or creams, washes, and just about anything that you can use water for when you want to add an herbal property to it.

If you are creating a water infusion to use as a beverage you can add Honey to it to sweeten the flavor. Do not add Sugar to your medicinal teas because Sugar has components in it that break down the medicinal properties of the plant and make it so that they will no longer provide the medicinal benefits you have created your infusion for. I like to add a little orange blossom Honey to my teas to sweeten and add a little bit of that citrus flavor.

Herbs for Water Infusions

Here is a list of a few herbs that are can be used as water infusions. This list is not at all extensive and I encourage you to find even more information. There are many plants that can be used for all types of infusions. Some have different properties that are drawn out better by water and other properties that may be drawn out better by alcohol or oil. Different parts of the plants are used in this way also.

Nettle is a very common herb that is used as a water infusion. Nettle contains many nutrients such as Vitamin A and Vitamin C, minerals including calcium, silicon, and Potassium chloride, protein, and dietary fiber. It is also considered a blood purifier but can have

16

a bitter taste. A Nettle infusion can be used as a hair rinse to encourage hair growth. It has been said that Nettle is also good for Anemia, Diabetes, Asthma and Allergies.

Red Clover is another herb that is good as a water infusion. Red Clover contains Vitamin C, Potassium, phosphorus, Magnesium, chromium and calcium. It is also reported to have diuretic, expectorant, antispasmodic and estrogenic properties. You will want to avoid Red Clover if you are taking any medications that might thin your blood.

Another commonly recommended herb for water infusions is Alfalfa. Alfalfa contains a lot of nutrients and, because of this, is a very good herb to take internally. It is high in Vitamin A, Vitamin K, several B vitamins as wells as iron, calcium, Magnesium, sulfur, phosphorus, sodium and Potassium. Alfalfa also helps you to absorb other plant nutrients and, therefore, can be used in conjunction with other herbs.

Chamomile infusions have antioxidants that may help prevent complications from Diabetes and stunt the growth of cancer cells. It is also relaxing and can help with stomach problems. Chamomile is antifungal, soothing and cleansing to the skin. Chamomile flowers are a good way to reduce frequent inflammation. An infusion of Chamomile flowers is especially recommended for the fragile skin around the eyes. Just take a couple of Chamomile tea bags, steep them in hot water, let them cool and place them over your eyes for several minutes.

Calendula (Calendula Officinalis), also known as Pot Marigold, is very healing, softening and soothing to the skin. It also has antifungal, anti-inflammatory, and antiseptic properties.

Elder Flower is a gentle cleanser, toner, and astringent. It can be helpful when dealing with colds and fevers as well. Elder Flower also helps reduce inflammation.

Rosemary is antiseptic and toning. It also improves blood circulation and has anti-inflammatory properties.

Thyme is a strong antibacterial herb. It can be used as a skin wash for acne. You can combine it with Calendula to soothe and heal your skin.

Many herbs contain vital nutrients that can be extracted in a water infusion and taken internally. I can't stress enough the need for you do your research to find out what herb(s) to use and for what reasons.

Bath "Teas"

What is a bath tea? A bath tea is when you make an herbal water infusion and add it to a bath in order to soak the properties of the herbs into your skin and/or breathe in the aromatic scents.

In order to make a bath tea you just use the methods that were discussed earlier in this chapter. You'll want to make a large batch and then add it to your bath water.

You will find some good bath tea recipes later on in this book but you can always experiment on your own.

Another way to make a bath tea is to get a large bath tea bag that has drawstrings and put the herbs into the bag. Make sure to tie it off well unless you want herbs floating around in your bath water and sticking to your body when you get out. You can hang the bag from your faucet and allow the hot water to run through it or you can draw a very hot bath and throw the bag into the water to steep.

Facial Steams

Facial steams are great for your pores and can also help with sinus congestion.

In order to do a steam you will want to grab a bowl and a large towel. Make your herbal infusion and, while it is still hot and steaming, pour it into your bowl. Cover your head with the towel and lean down over the bowl. Make sure that the towel makes a tent that covers the bowl so the steam won't escape easily.

If you are using a steam to clear your sinuses, or to help you breathe, you will want to breathe in as deeply as possible.

If you are doing a cosmetic steam, just allow the steam to rise up and coat your skin.

Some really good herbs for a sinus congestion and/or chest congestion steam are Peppermint, Eucalyptus, whole Cloves and Mullein.

Herbs that can be used for a facial steam will depend on your skin type and what you're trying to accomplish. If you have oily skin you will want to use astringent herbs like Rosemary. If you have dry skin you'll want to use herbs that will moisturize and/or soften your skin such as Rose petals.

Remember to keep your face 5-10 inches away from the bowl so you don't burn yourself. If the steam gets too much for you, take a little break from being underneath the towel and then go back to it.

Oil Infusions

Infused oils should NOT be confused with essential oils. Essential oils are extremely concentrated and are sometimes combined with carrier oils like the ones used in our infusions.

True essential oils are strictly oils extracted from the plant material and contain no carrier oils. Many should not be used internally or applied directly to the skin. Many companies that you find in some craft stores will try to sell an "essential oil" that is actually fragrance oil (often an oil infused with an artificial fragrance) or essential oil diluted in carrier oil (creating an infused oil) to make it more affordable. Essential oils do not go rancid but should still be stored in a cool, dark place to maintain their potency. They can lose their therapeutic qualities over time. Carrier oils will go rancid and should also be stored in a cool, dark place.

When making oil infusions you can use lots of different oils. My favorite is Extra Virgin Olive Oil but you can use Olive Oil, Canola Oil, Sunflower Oil, Sesame Oil, Almond Oil, Avocado Oil, Jojoba Oil or a plethora of other oils.

Different oils have all different properties when applied to the skin. Some, like Almond oil, soak into the skin more readily than others and so shouldn't be used for massage oils or anything that requires the oil remain on top of the skin for a length of time. Other oils, like

22

Olive Oil, are good for this purpose because they take a little longer to be absorbed.

These oils also have different shelf lives. Please check to see what the shelf life is of the particular oil that you're using so that you can store it properly. Extra Virgin Olive Oil, stored in a unopened container, can last three years (though the average shelf life is about 2 years, as seen in the list on the next page). Keeping the oils away from light, heat and ail will help to extend their shelf lives.

Here is a list of different oils you might like to use and their average shelf life:

Almond Oil ~ 1 year
Avocado Oil ~ 1 year
Jojoba Oil ~ 2+ years
Olive Oil ~ 2 years
Sesame Oil ~ 1 year
Sunflower Oil ~ 1 year

You can combine different oils for their different properties also. Some of the oil with a longer shelf life can help to extend the shelf life of the ones that don't last quite as long.

Almond oil, or Sweet Almond Oil, soaks into the skin pretty quickly and is better used for things that you don't need to stay on top of the skin for an extended length of time. It is a thin oil that has a slight nutty aroma. It is a good oil to use for lip balms (which are a form of salve).

Avocado Oil has lots of vitamins A, D and E. It also contains protein and amino acids. All of these are great for mature skin. It is a good nourishing oil for both skin and hair. It is a thick oil and can leave a waxy coat on the skin. It is usually mixed with another oil when used for skin care. Do not refrigerate.

Jojoba Oil is a good choice for people with acne prone skin. It is technically a wax but is very close in composition to our skin's natural oils. It is also said to have anti-inflammatory properties. It is good for all skin types and readily absorbed.

Olive Oil is very mild and moisturizing. I like to use Extra Virgin Olive Oil for a lot of what I do. It's affordable and works well for lotions, creams and massage oils. The downside of using Olive Oil is that it does have a fragrance to it which can overpower other scents. It can also cause an allergic reaction in some people.

Sesame Oil, also known as Sesame Seed Oil, is a thick oil with a slight aroma and can have a dark color. It is best blended with other oils and very good for massage. It is also said to have anti-inflammatory properties and is good for all skin types.

Sunflower Oil is a good, all-purpose oil. Try to get unrefined if possible. It is a thin oil with a faint, sweet scent. It can be almost odorless. It is great for those who are allergic to nuts or who may have delicate skin. It is rich in vitamins and minerals.

If any of your carrier oils develop a strong bitter aroma they have gone rancid and should be disposed of. The shelf lives will vary quite a bit based on how an oil was processed and how it has been stored.

As with anything that you are going to put on or in your body, you want to make sure that there are no allergies or dietary concerns with the oils that you use.

It is advised to use dried herbs when you are making herbal infused oils. The reason for this, in the oil infusion, is because fresh herbs contain moisture that puts your oil at greater risk for bacterial growth and spoilage.

Solar Oil Infusions

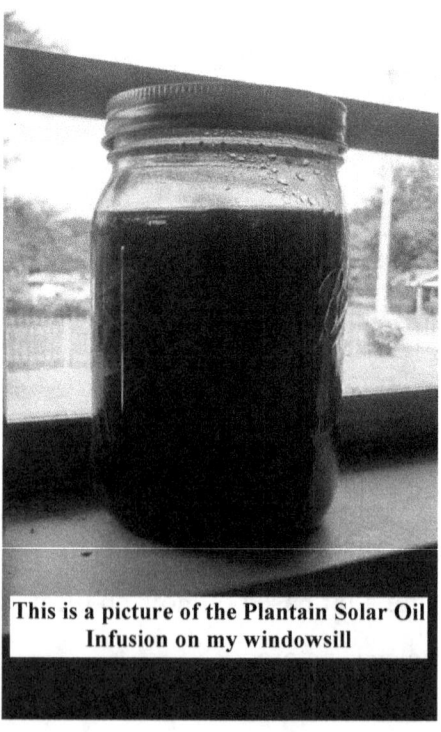

This is a picture of the Plantain Solar Oil Infusion on my windowsill

To make a solar infusion (also known as a cold infusion) with oil you will want to use the same process as the solar water infusion. I will include those steps again here in case you missed the first part.

26

A solar infusion uses the heat of the sun to warm the oils so that they will extract what is needed out of the plants. To do this you take a clean, sterile jar, fill it with plant material, cover the plant material in the oil of your choice, get as much air bubbles out as you can (you can use a cHopstick or something similar to stir around the plant material and release the air pockets), seal with a clean, sterile lid and sit on a sunny, warm windowsill for a 2-4 weeks depending on the weather. Put a label on the jar with all of the information you will need: the name of the herb you are using, the type of infusion (water, oil, etc.), the date which you started the infusion and the date which the infusion should be ready to use.

Make sure that, when you pour the oil over the herbs, you fill it until the oil reaches just over the top of the herbs. All of the plant material must be covered to help avoid any growth of bacteria or fungi. At least once every day you will want to turn or shake your bottle and make sure that the plant material is still covered by the oil. If you use dry herbs the plant material may swell as it becomes rehydrated.

After the appropriate amount of time, you will want to remove the jar from its sunny location and strain the plant material from the liquid using cheesecloth, a coffee filter, a French Press, or any other way you feel comfortable. You want to make sure that you have been able to remove any of the particles left over from the plant material itself. You can then compost your leftover plant material and store your infusion or use it.

If you would like to make a stronger concentration of oil, you can put more herbs in the jar and add the already infused oil to them and continue to do so until it is as concentrated as you would like.

If you want to add a natural preservative to your infused oils you can use some Vitamin E oil or some Grapefruit Seed Extract. You should only need a very small amount of either depending on the amount of infusion you are adding the preservative to.

The Stove or Fire Method

If you want to infuse your oils on a stove or over a fire you will want to place your plant material into a pot and cover it with oil. Place the pot over the fire (or on the burner). Be very careful with this method because you could end up cooking the herbs. You don't want to cook them; you just want to infuse the oil with the essences of the herbs. Place the pot on the lowest heat setting possible. You want to heat the oil enough to infuse the herbs but you don't want to fry them. Let the herbs infuse for about 3 hours but keep an eye on them to make sure the heat is not too high. When they are thoroughly infused remove them from the heat and allow the infusion to cool off. Once it's cool you can strain out the plant material. At this time you can add in the Vitamin E oil or Grapefruit Seed Extract.

Another stove or fire method is done by using a double boiler or bain-marie. There is less chance of frying your plant material if you use this method. You can either buy a double boiler or make one yourself.

Merriam-Webster defines a bain-marie as this "a cooking utensil containing heated water in which food in smaller pots is cooked — compare double boiler". To make a double boiler you will need a glass or ceramic bowl that will fit in a pot. I like to use a glass bowl that's edges sit on the edge of the large pot. You will then fill the large pot about halfway with water and place the glass bowl in the pot. It should rest on top of or above the water. Place the plant material inside the bowl and then pour the oil over it. Turn on the heat as you did in the first method and allow it to steep for the same amount of time. The water acts as a barrier to keep the plant material from frying in the oil, using indirect heat, but it still needs to be watched carefully.

Again, remove the infusion from the heat and allow it to cool before straining it. You can then add your preservative.

The Slow Cooker Method

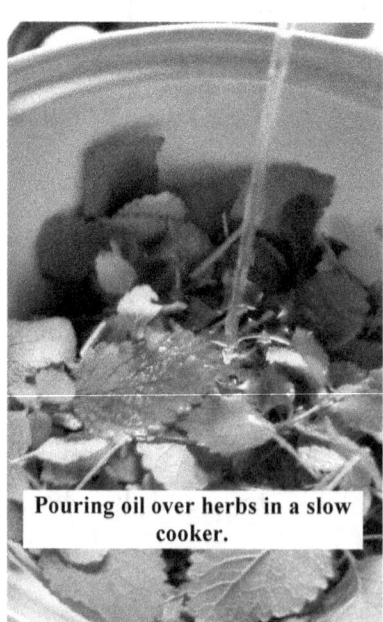

Pouring oil over herbs in a slow cooker.

The slow cooker method is my preferred method of infusing oils. It is a great method for those who may be doing many things at once. It is still possible to fry your plant material using this method though it is less likely.

I use a small two quart slow cooker for this particular method. It has a "warm" setting and makes the oil in good sized batches. It is basically the same formula. You place your plant material in the bottom of the slow cooker and cover it with the oil. If your slow cooker has a "warm" setting you will want to use that. If your slow cooker doesn't have a "warm" setting you will want to place it on the lowest setting possible. I have seen a very small accessory for the slow cooker called a "Little Dipper" that could possibly be used for this purpose also though I have not tried it myself.

Lemon Balm after infusing in oil in the slow cooker.

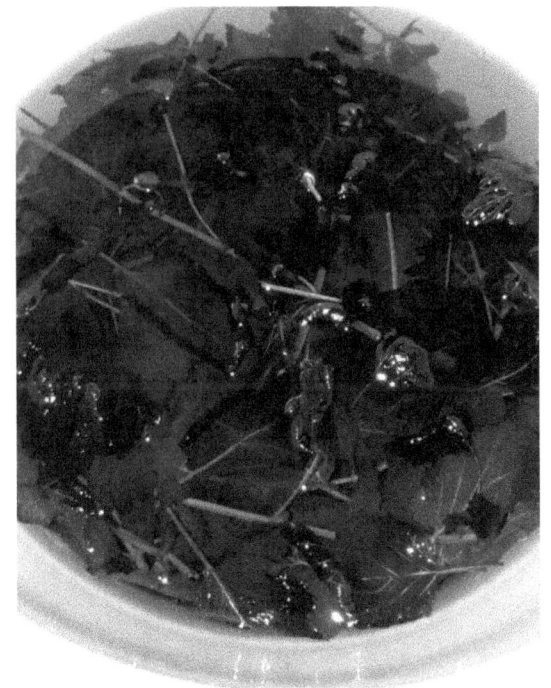

You can leave your plant material in the slow cooker for a few hours (usually around two to four) but make sure to check on it periodically.

When ready, turn off your slow cooker and allow the infusion to cool before straining.

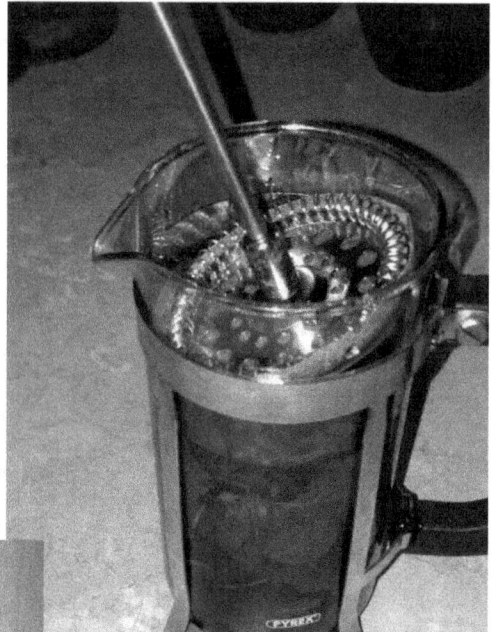

You can make your oil stronger and more concentrated by using the same method as

This is where I am starting to press the filter of the French Press down to strain the herbs from the infused oil.

This is when I placed the infused oil and herbs into the French Press.

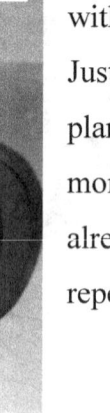

with the water infusions. Just strain the oil from the plant material and add more plant material to the already infused oil and repeat whatever process you have used to infuse the oil the first time.

Here you can see the filter all the way at the bottom of the press. The clear, strained liquid is above the filter.

Oil infusions can be used in foods (as a marinade or salad dressing), made into lotions, creams, salves, cleaning products and massage and/or body oils. There are a plethora of uses for infused oils. Make sure to store them in a cool, dark place. Using a brown or cobalt blue storage bottle or jar can extend their shelf life also.

Pouring the strained oil into a storage jar for later use.

Honey Infusions

Honey, by itself, is great for your body and skin. By infusing your Honey with herbs you can add to its natural benefits. Some studies have shown that Honey is even better than over-the-counter cough medicines!

When making a Honey infusion I would suggest that you get raw organic Honey for the best possible results. Using local Honey can add an even better component to your end product.

You can make a Honey infusion by pouring the Honey over the plant material and allowing it to steep using the solar infusion method for several weeks (usually around 6) or months. You don't want to use heat to infuse the Honey because it can damage the beneficial properties within the Honey itself.

Honey has antibacterial properties all on its own and so it doesn't need a preservative but make sure that all of the plant material is covered by the Honey. There have even been jars of Honey found in ancient Egyptian tombs that have still not gone rancid.

Honey infusions are more difficult to strain but it can be done. You can heat your Honey very slightly by sitting it in a jar of warm water in order to make it more liquid so that it will strain more readily.

Honey infusions can be used as medicinal syrups, lozenges, sweeteners for tea or coffee, glazes for meat, spread on toast but can also be used for external applications to the skin.

Some herbs that are commonly used for flavors in Honey are Rose petals, Chamomile, Lemon Balm, Basil, Ginger, Sage, Peppermint, Cinnamon, Vanilla, Star Anise, Rosemary, Thyme and Lavender.

Do not give Honey to children under 1 year of age. For a child that young Honey is dangerous in that it can cause the child to develop botulism which can cause paralysis and even death. Older children and adults are not harmed by this because of the large number of beneficial bacteria within our intestines.

How to Make Herbal Syrups

To make herbal syrups you will want to combine approximately 2 ounces of herbs with 1 quart of water in your pot. Begin simmering the mixture over low heat and reduce the liquid down to 1 pint (or about half). Strain the herbs and pour the liquid back into the pot. Add 1 cup of Honey per pint of liquid. Warm the Honey and water infusion just enough to blend them together. Do not cook it any longer than necessary or on higher heat so you don't destroy the healing properties of the Honey. You can then pour your syrup into a bottle or jar, label it and refrigerate it.

Good herbs to use to make syrups are Horehound (for coughs), Echinacea (for immune system boosting), Licorice Root (not the candy), Ginger, Valerian (for relaxation), Elderberry (for coughs), Cinnamon and whole Cloves.

Adults can take 1 tablespoon every hour and children can be given 1 teaspoon depending on their weight and age.

Decoctions

What is a decoction? A decoction is what you get when you boil the heartier parts of a plant (stems, bark, roots, some berries and seeds) making it another type of water infusion.

When you make a decoction using stems or roots you will want to chop the plant material up before you boil it. With barks, seeds and berries you may need to soak them in water for several hours before you boil them. Seeds and berries may need to be crushed first also.

When you are getting ready to make your decoction place your plant material in cold water and raise the heat gradually. I like to use the double boiler method for this so that the metal from my pot doesn't cause a reaction.

Once the water has reached the boiling point you want to reduce the heat to a simmer and allow it to do so for around thirty minutes to an hour or more depending on the density of the plant material you're using.

Syrups

To make a syrup you will use your water decoction or infusion and combine it with Honey. To do this you will make your decoction and keep it on the heat until the liquid is reduced to half of its original amount. If you are using a pint (about two cups) of concentrated decoction you will want to add one cup of raw Honey. Strain your decoction/infusion, compost the herbs, return the liquid back to the pot and add in your Honey. You then want to heat the mixture very slightly, while stirring, to combine all of the ingredients. This is great for herbs like Elderberry, Wild Cherry Bark, Valerian root and Horehound. Make sure to not heat it very long or very high. Heat will kill the beneficial aspects of the Honey. When everything is combined you will want to pour your newly made syrup into a bottle, label it and stick it in the refrigerator. The Honey in the syrup will help to preserve it as Honey does not go bad, however, keep an eye on it and if it begins to smell off or has any mold growth or anything that may give you a sense that the syrup has gone bad then discard it and make another if needed.

Decoctions are most often used when making syrups because the flavors of the sturdier parts of the plants can have a very strong and sometimes bitter taste. The Honey adds sweetness to the syrup and therefore makes it easier to take.

How to make Infusions and Decoctions by Starr Morgayne

Recipes

Herbal Hair Rinses

When making an herbal hair rinse you can use just an herbal water infusion or you can add some apple cider vinegar to it in order to remove buildup and residue. It also adds shine to the hair and improves circulation to the scalp.

There are a couple of different ways to use an herbal hair rinse. You can shampoo and rinse your hair first. Then you can either put it in a spray bottle, spray it onto your hair and massage it into your scalp or you can take two large bowls and pour the rinse from one bowl over your hair and into the other bowl. Then repeat the process by switching the bowls. You can switch the bowls several times. Make sure to avoid your eyes when using either of these procedures.

Most of these hair rinses do not have to be rinsed out. The smell of the vinegar will go away quickly so you don't have to worry about stinking like vinegar all day.

You can also use herbal water infusions to slightly color your hair. Some herbs, such as Rosemary or Sage, will darken your hair. To lighten your hair you can add Chamomile or citrus. Lavender and Tea Tree are good for dandruff.

Rosemary Peppermint Hair Rinse

1 part Rosemary
1 part Peppermint
3 parts water
2 parts Apple Cider Vinegar
Essential Oils (optional)

Rosemary cleanses the hair and can stimulate hair growth by increasing the circulation to the scalp. Peppermint helps to prevent hair from thinning.

In order to create this hair rinse you will want to combine chopped Rosemary and Peppermint leaves with the water. The size of the "parts" that you use will depend on the length of your hair. Heat the herbs and water to make an infusion.

After your infusion has steeped, allow it to cool and strain it. You can then add the apple cider vinegar to it.

Also, if you wish, you can add a few drops of essential oils at this time.

Vinegar Herb Dandruff Rinse

2 cups water
½ cup apple cider vinegar
2 Tbsp Rosemary
2 Tbsp Sage
1 Tbsp Nettle
5 drops each Tea**Error! Bookmark not defined.** Tree Oil, Rosemary essential oil and Lavender essential oil

Heat the water to point where it is just starting to boil. Remove it from the heat and add in the herbs. Steep the herbs for approximately two hours.

When the herbs are finished steeping, strain them through a coffee filter or some cheesecloth. I like to take either my coffee filter or cheesecloth and put them in a metal strainer over a bowl. When I'm straining the herbs out then I can fold the cloth over and put gentle pressure on it to make sure I'm getting everything out. When I'm finished I can throw the whole bundle (I use natural coffee filters) into the compost bucket. It's a great way to recycle.

Once you have the liquid strained from the herbs you'll then add in the essential oils and the apple cider vinegar and stir to mix everything together. You'll want to apply this to clean, damp hair (Make sure the hair is damp and not sopping wet) and massage it in for about two to three minutes. After the massage you'll then want to rinse with cool water.

Medicinal Oil Infusions

Here are a couple of the most common oil infusions that I use around my own home.

Clove Toothache Oil

I normally make this using Clove Essential Oil but you could also use whole Cloves and infuse them into the oil.

2 drops Clove Essential Oil
1 Tablespoon Olive Oil (or another oil with a mild taste)

Combine the ingredients and apply to sore gums. The Clove Oil acts as an analgesic and will soothe the pain. This can even be used on a teething infant. Reapply as necessary.

Mullein and Garlic Ear Oil

1 part Mullein flowers
1 part Garlic Cloves, minced

Mullein flowers can be collected as they appear on the tall stalk of the plant. I usually put them in a brown paper bag to dry. We get quite a bit of them here because my yard is filled with Mullein plants.

When you have enough dry Mullein flowers you will want to combine them with fresh, crushed or minced garlic Cloves.

Combine the herbs with oil and heat using whatever method of oil infusing you would like. Strain the oil, add a natural preservative if you like and put it into a dark colored jar with a dropper lid. Label it and keep it in your medicine cabinet for those times when someone may develop a mild earache or infection.

To apply the oil just put a couple of drops into the ear and then gently place a cotton ball at the opening of the ear to keep the oil from dripping out.

Teas

If you like to drink them, teas can be a very good way to get the medicinal qualities of many herbs into your system. You can use Honey, preferably raw and organic, to sweeten the taste of most teas.

Restful Sleep Tea

1 part Chamomile flowers
1 part Lemon Peel (without the pith or white part)
1 part Mint leaves

Pour hot water over approximately 1 ½ teaspoons of plant material and allow to steep for 5-10 minutes. Drink right before bed.

PMS Tea

2 parts Nettle leaves
1 part Lemon Verbena
1 part Lemon Balm

Pour hot water over approximately 1 ½ teaspoons of plant material and allow it to steep for 15-20 minutes. You can drink one or two cups a day during the week before you begin your menstrual cycle.

Cheer Up Tea

¼ Cup dried Chamomile flowers
¼ Cup dried Calendula (Pot Marigold) petals
1/8 C dried Peppermint leaves
1 tbsp grated Lemon Peel
½ tbsp whole Cloves
Honey to taste

When you want to make this tea take 1 ½ teaspoons of this mixture of herbs and cover them with 1 cup of hot water. Allow it to steep for 5-10 minutes. Strain it and sweeten it with Honey if you like.

I made up a bunch of this and gave it to a friend of mine who was battling Depression. She said that it helped her immensely.

Women's Tea Blend

1 part Nettle
1 part Raspberry Leaves
1 part Red Clover blossoms
Honey to taste

Pour hot water over approximately 1 ½ teaspoons of plant material and allow it to steep for 15-20 minutes. The combination of these plants is very good for a woman's hormonal issues.

Calming Bath Tea

2 parts Lavender
2 parts Chamomile
1 part Hops
1 part Rosebuds

Pour boiling water over herbs and allow them to steep for 10-15 minutes. For a bath tea you can either strain the plant material out or leave it in. After the tea has steeped for long enough, pour it into your already drawn bath. Relax in your bath and breathe in the wonderful aroma of these soothing herbs.

Sinus Bath Tea

2 parts Eucalyptus
2 parts Peppermint
1 part whole Cloves

Pour boiling water over herbs and allow them to steep for 10-15 minutes. For a bath tea you can either strain the plant material out or leave it in. After the tea has steeped for long enough, pour it into your already drawn bath. Relax in your bath and breathe in the wonderful aroma of these soothing herbs. This bath tea should help to clear some of your sinus congestion.

Syrups

Elderberry Cough Syrup

2 Cups water
1 Cup fresh Elderberries or ½ C dried Elderberries
1 Cup raw Honey

Make a decoction of the berries by putting them in a pot

with the water and bringing them to a boil. Turn down the heat and allow them to simmer for about 30 minutes stirring occasionally. When it's done you'll want to strain the mixture and allow it to cool a bit. When it is still somewhat warm go ahead and add the Honey. Make sure it is not too hot though because you don't want to lose the beneficial properties of the Honey. Stir everything together well and pour it into your bottle or jar. Make sure to add a label.

You can also add other herbs if you want different properties such as Ginger or Mullein for congestion. You can also add other flavorings like Lemon or Cinnamon.

Horehound Cough Syrup

Rodale's Illustrated Encyclopedia of Herbs has a lovely recipe for making a Horehound cough syrup.

"Make an old-time cough remedy by mixing Horehound tea with Honey. Make an infusion by steeping 1 ounce of fresh or dried Horehound leaves in a pint of boiling water. Allow it to steep only 10 minutes. Strain off the leaves, then measure the quantity of liquid remaining. Add twice as much Honey as liquid, mix well, and bottle. To soothe a cough, take 1 teaspoon at a time, about 4 times a day!"

Afterword

Many people today are not only concerned about the environment but also about their own health and more conscious about what they are putting in and on their bodies.

We have come to be a society that tends to rely on synthetic chemicals. Many of these synthetic chemicals originate from natural sources. Unfortunately, these natural sources have been taken apart, studied and the components with the desired effect have been isolated. The reason that this is a bad thing is because that the plants these components come from contain other components that work in harmony with each other. When you have a drug that causes side effects the natural source that the drug was taken from probably has other things in it to counteract those side effects. Instead of using those natural sources to harmoniously heal ourselves we end up taking pill after pill to combat a disease or illness and then to combat the side effects that the first pill caused.

Because of the recent trend toward healing the earth and using more natural products, many companies have put out products that use buzz words like "organic" and "natural". The sad thing is that your basic consumer will probably assume that because these words are listed on the label it means that this is a good for the environment product or something that doesn't have harmful additives or chemicals. Sadly, this is not the case. If you look closely at the label you may find that the product you're looking at with "organic" on the label only has one ingredient in it that is actually organic. The rest of the ingredients may be the same as every other similar product on the shelf. The same goes for those products labeled "natural".

In my life I use a combination of Naturopathy (healing through food), herbalism (healing through herbs) and aromatherapy (healing through scent). I am not against using allopathic medicine (what we have come to know as "traditional" medicine) for severe issues and/or emergencies. In those areas, allopathic medicine excels. I am a firm believer in integrated medicine. Integrated medicine is using a combination of natural healing modalities as well as allopathic medicine.

I hope that through my writing I can inspire you to take your health more personally and discover the things that you can do to create a better self in a more natural and harmonious manner.

Glossary of Terms

Analgesic – An analgesic is something that reduces pain

Anemia – Anemia is a condition in which your blood has a lower than normal number of red blood cells often referred to as an iron deficiency.

Anti-inflammatory – An anti-inflammatory is something that decreases inflammation.

Antibacterial – An antibacterial is something that destroys or inhibits the growth of bacteria.

Antimicrobial – An antimicrobial destroys or inhibits the growth of micro-organisms

Antioxidant – An antioxidant is a substance that reduces the damage that oxygen does to the tissue, usually caused by free radicals which are chemicals that attack the molecules in your skin.

Antiseptic – An antiseptic helps to prevent infection and to get rid of disease causing organisms.

Antispasmodic – An antispasmodic is used to help control the spasms of an involuntary muscle.

Antitussive – An antitussive is something that prevents or relieves a cough.

Antiviral – Something that is antiviral kills or prevents a virus from multiplying.

Astringent – An astringent is something that tightens soft tissue in order to slow the flow of secretions.

Carminative – A carminative is something that relieves flatulence (gas).

Decoction – A decoction is a type of infusion made by boiling roots, barks, seeds, stems, berries or heartier parts of plants

Demulcent – A demulcent is something soothing. Demulcents are usually used to soothe and soften inflamed skin.

Diaphoretic – A diaphoretic is something that has the power to increase perspiration (sweating).

Diuretic – A diuretic is something that has the power to increase urination.

Emmenagogue – An emmenagogue is something that stimulates or increases menstrual flow.

Emollient – An emollient is something that softens and moisturizes the skin. It is usually found in the form of a lotion or thick liquid.

Emulsifier – An emulsifier is something that allows ingredients that do not normally mix well to blend together. Example: oil and water.

Emulsion – An emulsion is a mixture of two (usually) liquids that don't normally mix. Example: oil and water.

Exfoliant – An exfoliant is an abrasive used to scrub the skin in order to remove dead skin cells and increase circulation.

Expectorant – Merriam-Webster defines an expectorant as "an agent that promotes the discharge or expulsion of mucus from the respiratory tract; *broadly* : an antitussive agent"

Extract – When we use the word "extract" we can either be referring to the process of creating something or the product itself. Merriam-Webster defines this process as "to withdraw (as a juice or fraction) by physical or chemical process" or "to treat with a solvent so as to remove a soluble substance". The finished product is sometimes referred to as "an extract".

Fungicide – A fungicide, simply put, is something that kills fungi.

Germicide – A germicide is something that kills germs.

Glycerite – A glycerite is an infusion or tincture made using the syrupy liquid glycerine as the base. Using glycerine instead of alcohol provide an alcohol-free alternative for children and those who may have issues with alcohol.

Humectant – A humectant holds water or moisture (in this case it is something that will hold moisture to the skin)

Inflammation – The symptoms of inflammation are usually pain, swelling, redness and heat.

Infusion – In the case of this book an infusion is what you get when you use a liquid to pull the needed constituents of an herb out of the plant matter and into the liquid. Example: tea

Maceration – Technically, maceration is the preparation of an extract by soaking the containing material in an organic solvent. This would include infusions, decoctions, tinctures etc. but in herbal terms it has come to mean, a cold infusion of herbs in water, oil or vinegar.

Nervine – The word nervine refers to something that is used to calm the nerves. A couple of examples would be Lavender and Valerian.

Poultice – A poultice is usually a warm, wet mass that is applied externally. It is most often on or in between cloth and used for inflamed areas of the body.

Salve – Merriam-Webster's Online Dictionary defines a salve as "an unctuous adhesive substance for application to wounds or sores." My definition of a salve is a mixture of herb infused oil with either beeswax, hydrogenated vegetable oil (like Crisco), Coconut Oil, or a similar substance.

Sebaceous Gland – The sebaceous glands are small glands in the skin which secrete a lubricating oily matter (sebum) into the hair follicles to lubricate the skin and hair.

Sebum – The natural oil secreted onto our skin by our sebaceous glands is known as sebum.

Steeping – Steeping is the process used to make an infusion. You would cover your plant matter with hot liquid and let it steep by letting it sit for however long is needed.

Tincture – A tincture is what you get when you infuse alcohol with plant matter.

How to make Infusions and Decoctions by Starr Morgayne

Tools

Here is some information on some of the tools that you might like to have when you are making your own infusions and decoctions. You will want to make sure that you have separate items for making your medicinal preparations than you use for cooking because some of the ingredients you use may become absorbed by the tools and won't bode well for your cooking. If you are using essential oils remember that they can melt plastic.

Coffee Grinder ~ One of my favorite and most used tools is my coffee grinder. It is wonderful to use when I need to turn a dried herb into a powder.

Wooden Spoons ~ Wooden spoons are good for stirring your mixtures as they won't impart some of the impurities that using metal or plastic will. However, they can soak up smells and other components of what you are stirring them with.

Bowls ~ You'll need bowls to mix your ingredients. For some things you can use plastic bowls but for others you may want to use glass or ceramic.

Blender ~ A blender is good to have for making emulsions for lotions or creams. I have one blender for edible items and another for making my skin care products.

Cheesecloth ~ You can use this to make bath bags or tea bags. Cheesecloth can also be used for straining oils or other liquids through.

Coffee filters ~ Used for straining, similar to cheesecloth.

Double Boiler ~ In essence, this is two pans (or a pot and a glass bowl) put together. The one on the bottom has water in it. It is used to keep sensitive ingredients from getting too hot and burning. It is also known as a bain-marie.

Strainers ~ You can place cheesecloth or coffee filters within the strainer to strain the herb bits out of your infusions.

Measuring cups and spoons ~ You will need liquid measuring cups as well as those meant for solids.

Funnels ~ Funnels make filling bottles so much easier and a lot less messy. You will want to have several different sizes.

Mortar & Pestle ~ Every kitchen should have a mortar and pestle. It is good to use to grind up those things that you just can't get ground properly in a food processor or coffee grinder.

Pans ~ You can go with ceramic pans but you don't necessarily have to. Just remember that some metals may react adversely to some of the ingredients.

Bath Tea Bags ~ You don't necessarily have to have these but I love them. They're essentially large tea bags with drawstring closures. You can even use them to scrub yourself with or just hang them from your faucet for the water to flow through into the bath (after you've closed them and tied a knot in the drawstring at the opening of the bag and the end of the string). They're easily found at your local superstore or craft store. You can also sometimes substitute cheesecloth or even a wash cloth that is tied up around whatever you are using.

French Press ~ This is a somewhat fancy and completely optional item to have on hand. I like to use mine for straining oils and teas because I can squeeze out more of the infusion than I could with cheesecloth. The cheesecloth tends to soak up some of the infusion and can let small particles through.

Ingredients

Almond Oil, Sweet ~ Sweet Almond Oil (sometimes just called Almond Oil) is absorbed readily into the skin and makes a wonderful massage and carrier oil that is good for all skin types. It conditions, heals, revitalizes, smoothes and softens skin as well as being an emollient. One drawback is that it has a short shelf life.

Aloe Vera ~ Many of you are familiar with the Aloe Vera plant and its burn healing properties and its ability to help repair damaged tissue. Aloe Vera draws and holds oxygen to the skin which aids in the healing process. The gel from the leaf can be used but you can also find Aloe Vera juice in your local grocery store. It is soothing, softening, astringent and rejuvenating. It helps to draw out infections and heals skin irritations. It can also help to combat wrinkles. I like to use Aloe Vera juice instead of water when I make my lotions to give them an extra boost.

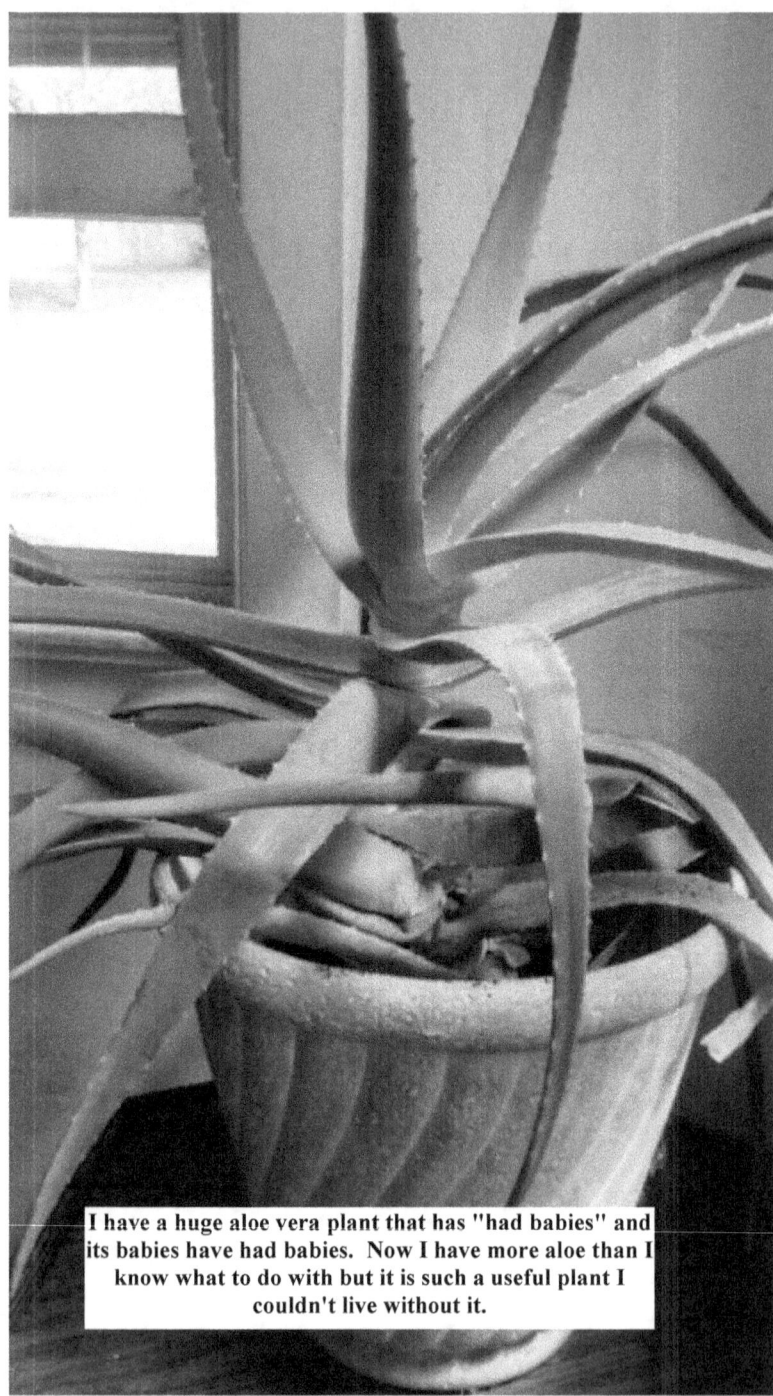

I have a huge aloe vera plant that has "had babies" and its babies have had babies. Now I have more aloe than I know what to do with but it is such a useful plant I couldn't live without it.

Apple Cider Vinegar ~ Apple Cider Vinegar is soothing and antiseptic. This valuable product helps to restore your skin's natural pH balance, relieve itchiness and is slightly astringent for those with normal to oily skin. It has been used for many years to help those afflicted with sunburn. Acetic acid is one of the main ingredients in Apple Cider Vinegar and has shown significant results for weight loss when used every day. It helps to create a more alkaline PH level within the system. It breaks up mucus within the body and cleanses the lymph nodes. It also helps relieve Candida because of the natural enzymes it contains.

Avocado ~ Avocado has nourishing and conditioning properties for both the skin and hair. The oil is used as an emollient. It is rich in proteins, minerals and vitamins and readily penetrates the skin. It is excellent for cracked or mature skin and heals, revitalizes and regenerates cells. Avocado Oil is excellent for face and massage oils. Avocadoes contain more Potassium than a banana and are also full of Vitamin D. The oils in the Avocado have been shown to reduce pain caused by Osteoarthritis. They have also been show to decrease "bad" cholesterol and increase "good" cholesterol.

71

Black Walnut ~ Black Walnut, specifically the hull, is often used for its antifungal properties as well as its astringency. It contains a high concentration of tannins which can also reduce pain and swelling. It is also

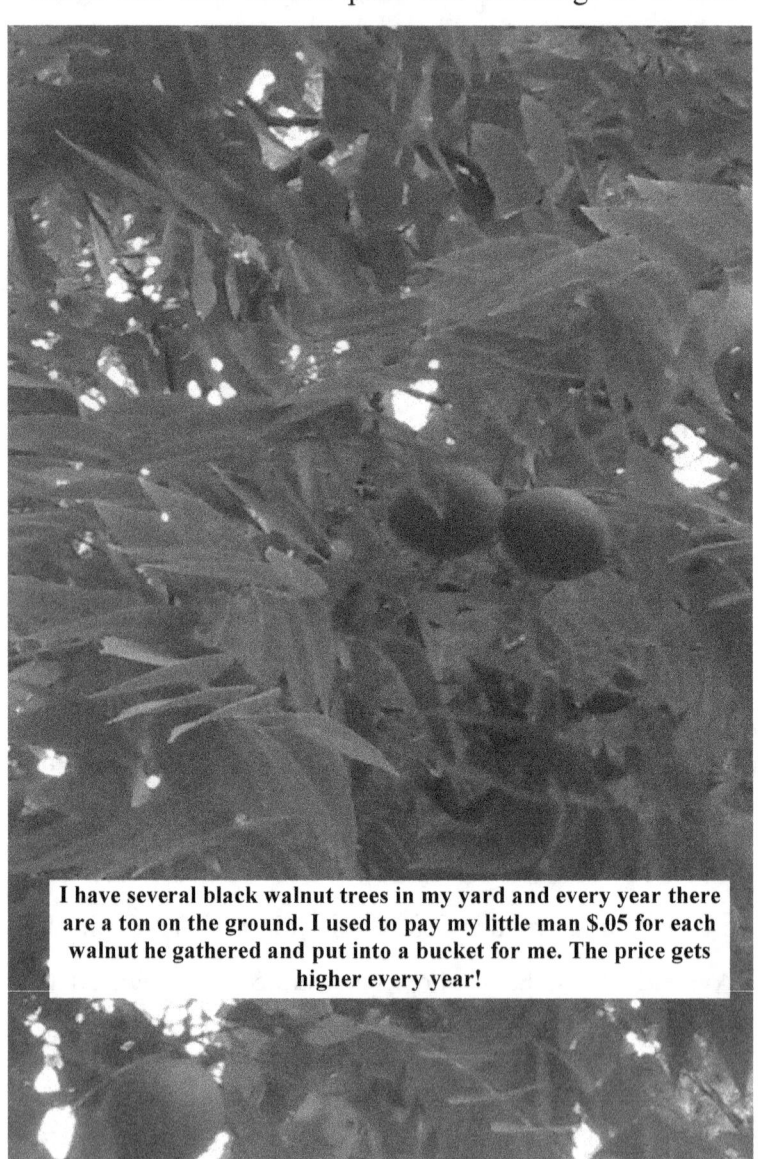

I have several black walnut trees in my yard and every year there are a ton on the ground. I used to pay my little man $.05 for each walnut he gathered and put into a bucket for me. The price gets higher every year!

antioxidant and antimicrobial. It is a natural laxative and a blood cleanser. If you've ever worked with Black Walnut Hull you are probably familiar with the fact that it can stain just about anything and has been used as a dye for centuries.

Burdock ~ Burdock is a plentiful (at least in my back yard) plant that has many different uses. You can use the leaves, roots and sometimes even the seeds. The roots are very bitter and can aid digestion, cleanse the liver, help absorb nutrients and eliminate waste. It can even help the liver's ability to metabolize hormones and therefore be used to treat hormonal imbalances such as estrogen dominance, endometriosis and Polycystic Ovarian Syndrome (PCOS). The root is sometimes sautéed with other vegetables in Oriental food dishes.

Calendula ~ Calendula (Calendula officinalis) is also known as Pot Marigold. It is very useful as a natural beauty tonic. It is anti-inflammatory, antiseptic, antifungal, antibacterial, cleansing, softening, smoothing as well as regenerative. It accelerates healing and can be used as a colorant. It is one of my favorite plants to use when making my own skin care products because it helps to tone and refresh the skin. It is useful in helping to prevent wrinkles and healing acne.

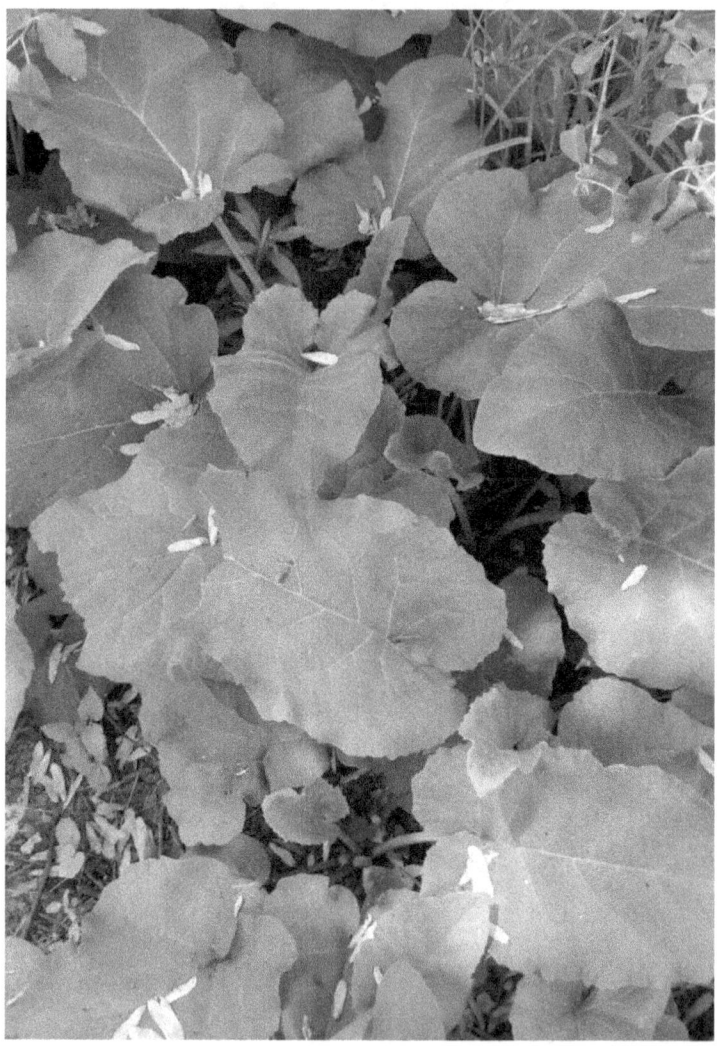

Here are the leaves of some Burdock plants in my yard. During their second year they will have long stalks with burrs at the end. This is how they got the name "Burdock".

Catnip ~ Catnip can be used in tea form to soothe and relax. It is even mild enough to give to small children. It is part of the Mint family and, as such, is said to help with digestive upsets in adults and to help with colic in children.

Chamomile, German ~ Chamomile tea is a great anti-inflammatory for pimples/zits/acne and is good for helping you relax and sleep. It is mildly astringent, diaphoretic, restorative and healing. Chamomile can also be used as a general anti-inflammatory and an antispasmodic.

Cinnamon ~ Cinnamon is antiseptic, astringent and stimulating. The powder can be used as an exfoliant but be careful because it can also be very irritating. Cinnamon has also been shown to lower the blood Sugar so it may be good for Diabetics. A popular way to take Cinnamon (other than on applesauce, oatmeal, or in a dessert) is to mix it with Honey and to eat a tablespoon of this infused syrup once a day. A study performed in Copenhagen found that this syrup helped with arthritis pains.

Clove ~ Cloves are antiseptic and their smell, usually brought out by using the essential oil, is used to calm and relieve stress. The oil is wonderful for toothaches as well. Whole Cloves (pictured below) are actually a flower bud.

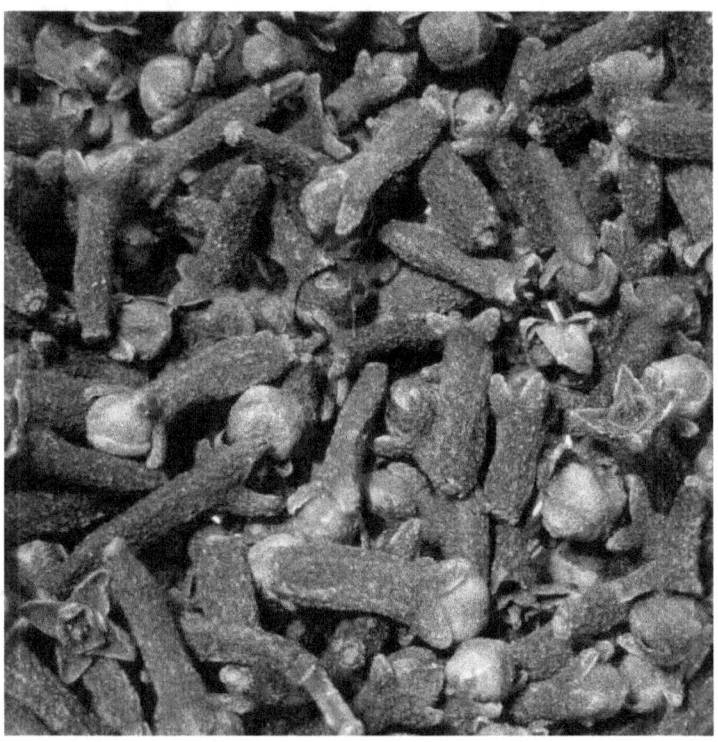

Clover, Red ~ Red Clover is astringent (due to tannins) and anti-inflammatory. It is often used in combinations created for women's health issues. It is said that a tea made from Red Clover is good for symptoms of menopause.

Clover, White ~ White Clover is very common in my area. It is a cousin to the Red Clover. The young flowers are very sweet and can be eaten raw. It was used medicinally by Native Americans to heal and cleanse boils and wounds as well as made into to tea for coughs, colds and fevers.

Comfrey ~ Comfrey is used to soothe and lubricate dry skin. It is also helpful in cell regeneration. The leaf can be used as a compress for swelling and bruising. I use it, infused in oil with Calendula petals, as a base for many of my healing lotions, creams and salves.

Dandelion ~ Dandelions are often thought of as a common "weed" but, then again, so are many other useful plants. It can be used for food as well as medicine. It has been touted as a heartburn remedy, a coffee substitute (by roasting the roots) and as a cure-all for just about everything. Dandelion leaves are rich in minerals and have been said to aid in fighting off Osteoporosis. It is said that drinking a tea made of the

Dandelion leaves can increase mobility and reduce stiffness. It is also thought to be most helpful for the liver for which it is a detoxifier and a strengthener.

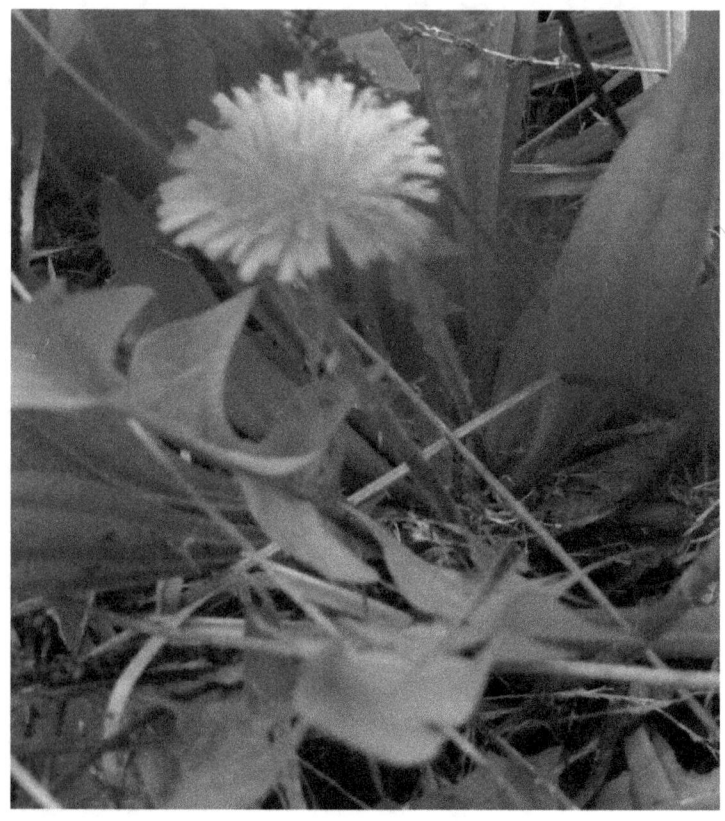

Echinacea ~ Echinacea, or Purple Coneflower, has long been used as an immune system booster. The most useful part of the plant is the root. You can make a decoction of it to drink or dry it and grind it into powder to make your own herbal capsules. You will want to make sure to use either Echinacea Purpura or Echinacea Angustifolia, as these are the most common medicinal forms of Echinacea.

Elderberry ~ Elderberry syrup is commonly used for colds and flu. Elderberry is another good herb that is used as an immune system stimulant. Elderberries are rich in Vitamin C and have antiviral properties. They also seem to have expectorant and astringent properties that can help reduce congestion and get rid of phlegm.

Eucalyptus ~ Eucalyptus is most commonly used externally as an inhalation and vapor rub to treat and relieve mucus congestion. It can help with bronchitis, colds, flu and sinusitis. As an oil infusion it can be used for bruises, sprains, strains and various muscle pains.

Fennel ~ Fennel has restorative, cleansing, detoxifying and antiseptic properties. It helps maintain the elasticity of the skin because of an estrogen-like substance it contains. All parts of the plant can be used. Hippocrates even suggested using Fennel tea to increase the flow of breast milk in nursing mothers.

Feverfew ~ Feverfew is a good herb to treat headaches and even migraines. It is usually combined with other herbs in a medicinal tea because it has a bitter taste. It is often mistaken for Chamomile. It has proven to be the most effective if taken as you feel the headache or migraine coming on. It is anti-inflammatory due to its ability to hinder the production of prostaglandins which are hormone-like substances that cause pain and inflammation. Some studies have found that the anti-inflammatory effects of this Feverfew are even greater than those achieved by NSAIDs (Nonsteroidal anti-inflammatory drugs) such as Ibuprofen or Naproxin.

Garlic ~ Garlic can, and should, be eaten as food but it can also be used as a medicinal herb. Garlic has been shown to mildly lower blood pressure by dilating or expanding blood vessels. It also helps prevent blood clots, reducing the risk of heart attack and stroke, by decreasing the stickiness of platelets. When platelets are too sticky, they form clumps that can adhere to artery walls and contribute to clogged arteries. There are studies that also show it is helpful in reducing the pain and inflammation of arthritis, reducing the size of some cancerous tumors, preventing some forms of cancer.

Garlic is also antibiotic, antiviral, antifungal and antibacterial.

Ginkgo Biloba ~ The "Biloba" part of the name Ginkgo Biloba refers to the leaves that have two "lobes". It is a very distinct and easy to recognize plant. Ginkgo is antioxidant and a circulation stimulant. Today, it is most commonly used to increase memory. It improves blood circulation by opening the blood vessels and making the blood less sticky.

Ginkgo has been used to regulate blood flow to the brain but has also been shown to protect nerve cells that have been damaged by Alzheimer's disease. It has even been shown to help in cases of glaucoma, macular degeneration, leg pain and other circulatory problems.

Glycerine ~ Glycerine (sometimes seen as Glycerin) is derived from vegetable or animal sources (I use vegetable glycerine myself) and is a wonderful moisturizer and skin cleanser that softens and lubricates. Vegetable glycerine is hypoallergenic and easily soluble in water. Vegetable glycerine has a long shelf life and a sweet taste which is why it is ideal to make medicinal syrups for children.

81

Green Tea ~ Green Tea has become popular in recent years because of its antioxidant properties. It is also popular belief that Green Tea has anti-aging properties. It can be used as a face rinse to tighten the pores.

Honey ~ Honey has many wonderful properties. It is antibacterial, emollient, moisturizing, nourishing, soothing and cleansing. It also promotes healing. In ancient times it was thought to be "the food of the Gods" and what made them immortal. The Romans believed that using Honey on your skin made you more attractive especially when mixed with Olive Oil. Honey is one of the best known humectants and is high in Potassium, therefore making it difficult for bacteria to survive in it. Also, if you want to sweeten your medicinal teas you should use Honey instead of Sugar. Sugar has components in it that break down the medicinal properties in the teas and make them no longer work.

Honey, on the other hand, does not and is healthier for you than Sugar as well. Try to get organic raw Honey for the best results.

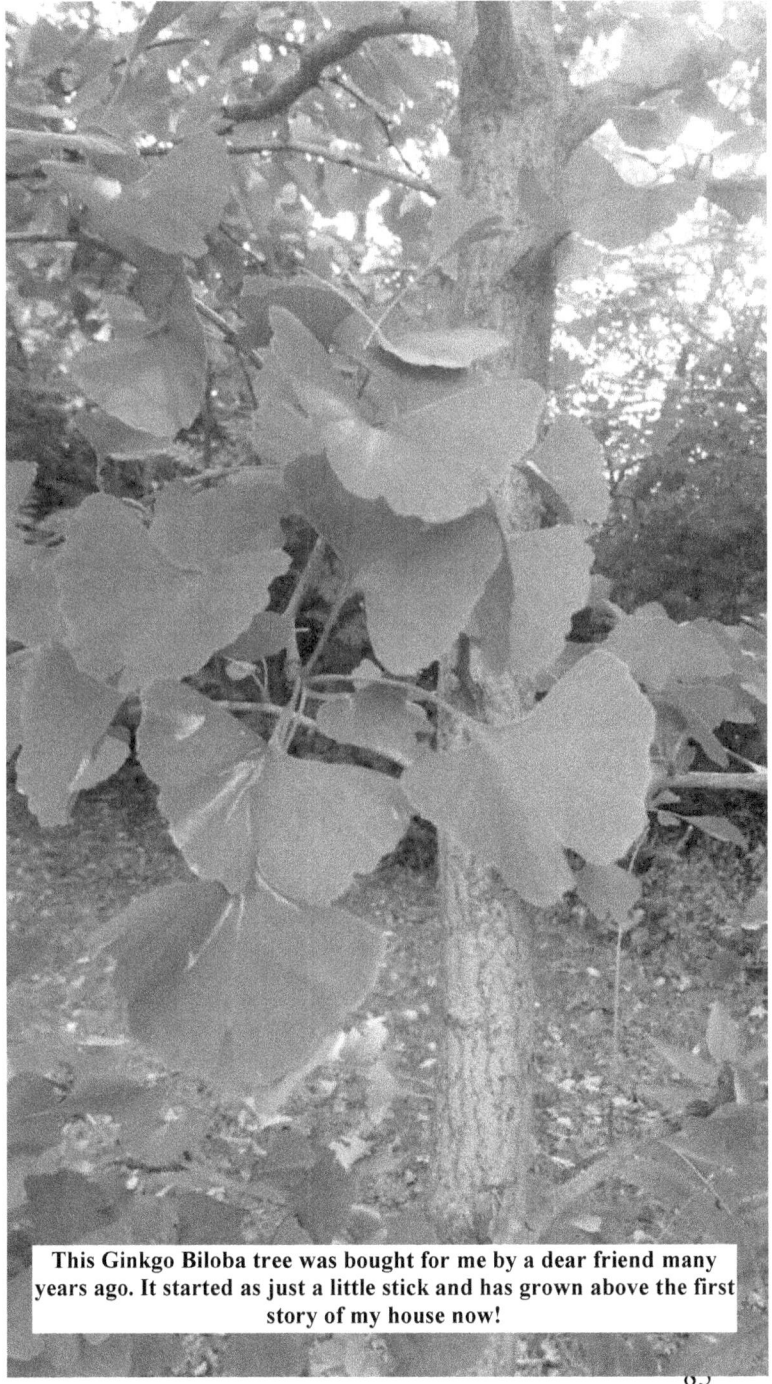

This Ginkgo Biloba tree was bought for me by a dear friend many years ago. It started as just a little stick and has grown above the first story of my house now!

Hops ~ Hops flowers are often used in a similar fashion to Valerian. They can be helpful for anxiety, insomnia, restlessness, tension, nervousness and irritability. Hops flowers are what gives beer its bitter flavor and are often used as a bitter tonic. They can lose their medicinal properties very quickly if exposed to light when stored.

Horehound ~ A good cough suppressant and expectorant is Horehound. It can be used as a syrup, a lozenge, a tea, etc to loosen phlegm from the chest. It contains a compound known as marrubiin which stimulates bronchial secretions and helps to break up congestion. It has been used for generations as a cure for children's cough, cold and croup. My grandmother used to tell me that when she was a little girl she loved eating Horehound candies. It may also be used to treat a mild upset stomach in children.

Jojoba Oil ~ Jojoba is very similar to the natural oil (known as sebum) that is secreted by your skin daily. Because of this, it is easily absorbed by the skin. Jojoba is a natural moisturizer and helps with renewal of skin cells. It also has antioxidant properties and is great for treating acne and problems such as eczema, psoriasis and dry skin.

Lavender ~ Lavender is one of my most favorite herbs. It is one of the few essential oils you can use neat (by itself, without diluting in a carrier oil) on the skin. It has so many wonderful properties as well; anti-inflammatory, antibacterial, antiseptic, balancing, relaxing, soothing. It helps both dry and oily skin by helping to normalize secretions from the sebaceous glands. It also stimulates growth of new cells. It can be used to repel insects as well as to calm yourself and reduce stress. Lavender can also help with sinus issues and headaches. If you are having trouble with either one take a couple drops of Lavender oil and put them on your temples and just under your eyes around the top of your cheek bones. This should help clear up the issue in no time.

Lemon ~ Lemon has antiseptic, rejuvenating, stimulating, astringent and mild bleaching properties. It also helps to restore the natural acid balance of the skin because it contains Citric Acid which is an AHA or alpha hydroxy acid and BHA or beta hydroxy acid.

Citric Acid also kills bacteria on the skin. Be careful though because citrus oils may irritate sensitive skins and cause photosensitivity (increased sensitivity to sunlight). Also, don't use on sore or irritated skin. The scent of Lemon is used in aromatherapy for its uplifting and refreshing effects.

Lemon Balm ~ Also known as Bee Balm or Melissa (its Latin name is Melissa Officinalis), Lemon Balm is part of the Mint family and is said to be antiviral. Studies have shown that putting a salve of Lemon Balm on herpes sores can make a huge difference in healing them.

Lemon Balm has also been used for digestive issues such as bloating, flatulence (gas), vomiting as well as menstrual cramps, headache, anxiety, restlessness, sleep disorders, ADHD, high blood pressure, sores and insect bites.

Due to its strong Lemon smell, Lemon Balm is excellent for adding to insect repellent recipes.

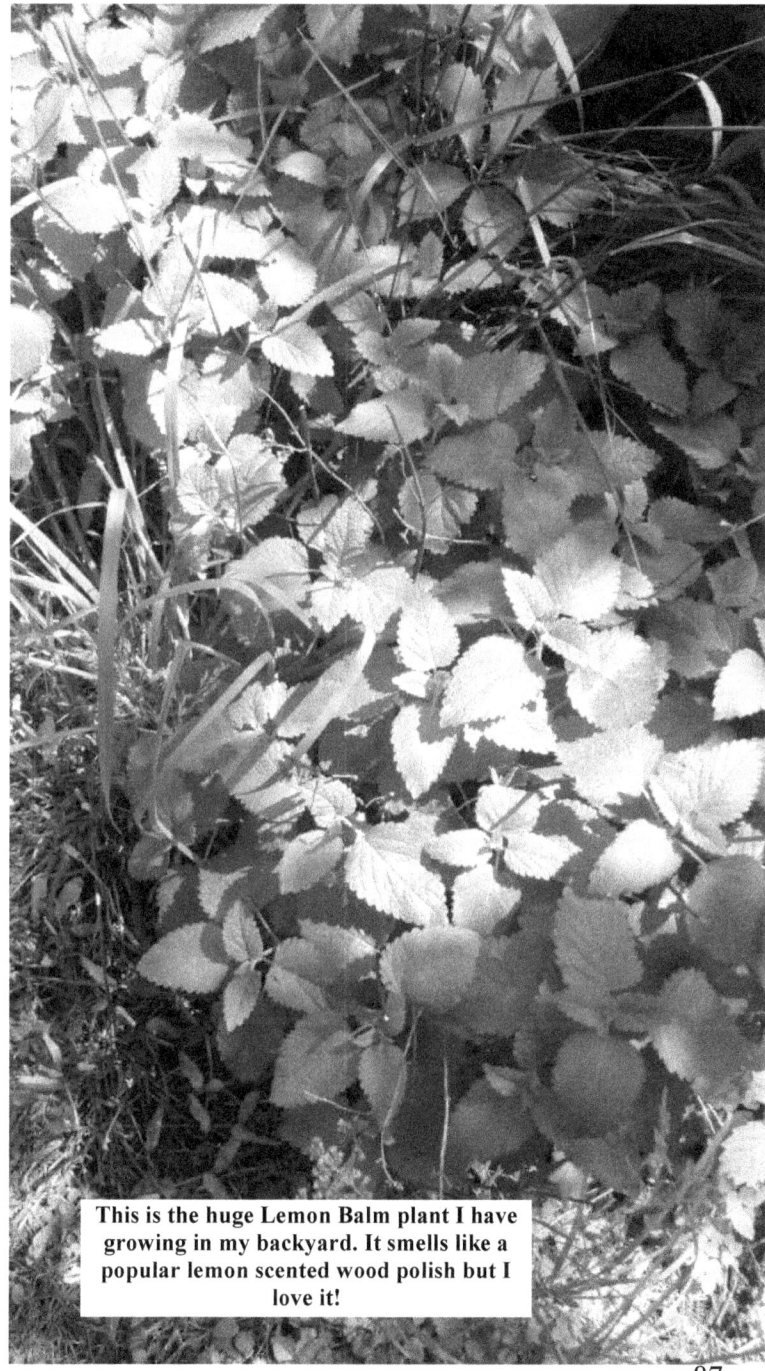

This is the huge Lemon Balm plant I have growing in my backyard. It smells like a popular lemon scented wood polish but I love it!

Lemon Verbena ~ Lemon Verbena, sometimes called Vervain, has been used for indigestion, gas, diarrhea, constipation, joint pain, insomnia, colds, fevers and varicose veins. It is most commonly used as a flavoring agent due to its extremely strong Lemony smell.

Lemongrass ~ Lemongrass is said to be antifungal, analgesic, astringent and can increase circulation.

Mint ~ Members of the Mint family tend to be naturally astringent as well as refreshing. They are good to use to boost your mood or wake you up. Some members of the Mint family are Spearmint, Peppermint, Wintergreen and Catnip.

Mullein ~ The Mullein plant is very good for problems related to breathing and congestion. You can drink Mullein tea to break up the mucus that clogs the lungs. You can also combine Mullein with garlic in an oil infusion to make a wonderful oil for ear infections. In ancient times Mullein leaves were used as diapering material for infants, menstrual pads for women and toilet tissue due to their softness.

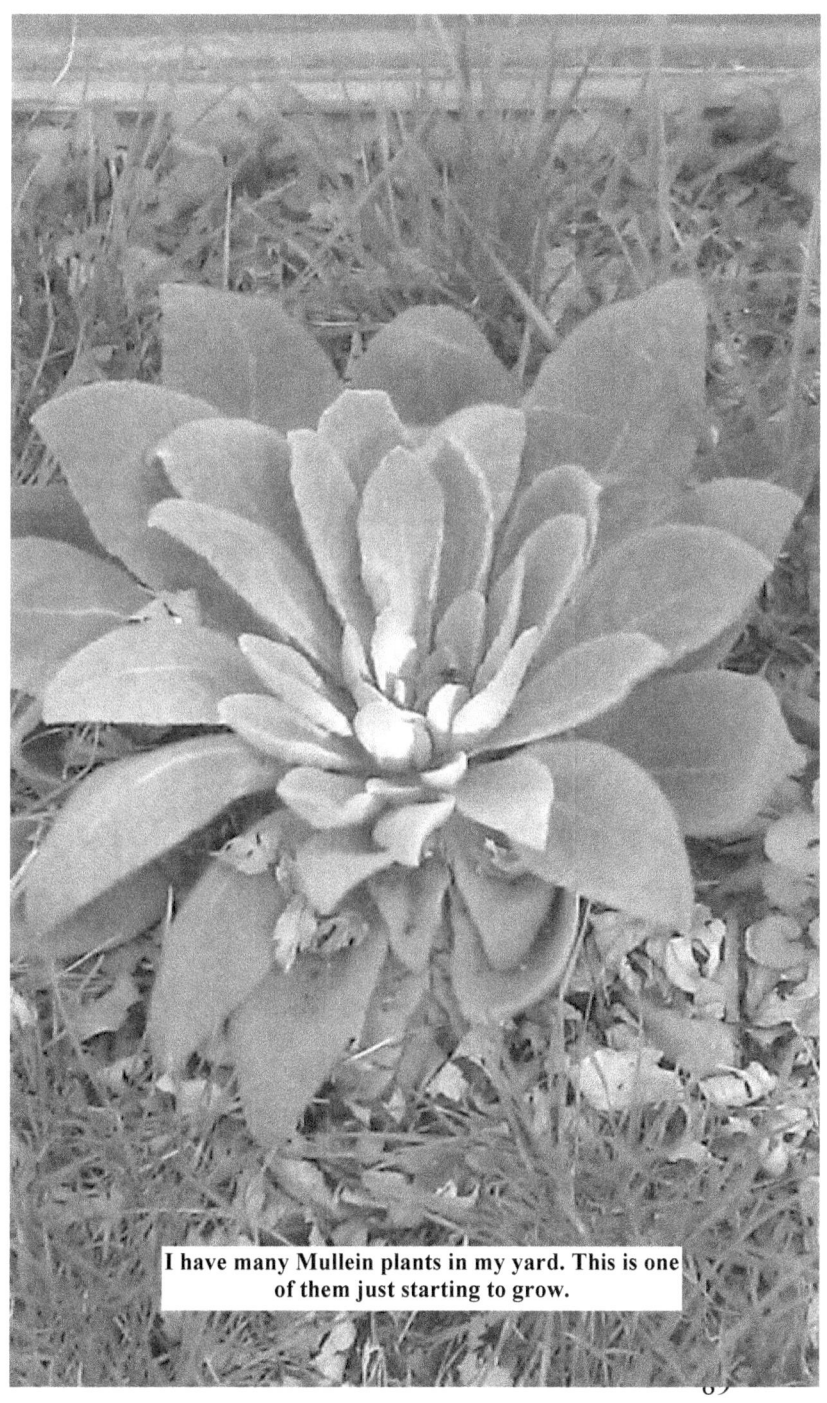

I have many Mullein plants in my yard. This is one of them just starting to grow.

Nettle ~ Nettle leaf, also known as Stinging Nettle, is best used fresh. It is full of nutrients and is often used to help with women's hormonal imbalances. You can make it into a tea or you can dry it and make your own herbal capsules. It is said to stimulate hair growth and is good for bronchial and asthmatic issues. I have heard of using the whole plant for arthritis pains by brushing the leaves over the afflicted area.

Olive Oil ~ Olive Oil is often used as an emollient and it attracts moisture to the skin. It has a long shelf life and blends well with other oils. I like to use Extra Virgin Olive Oil. You can often store Olive Oil, without refrigeration, for up to a year. It is especially good for dry skin and makes and excellent conditioner for nails and hair.

Onion ~ Onions are antibacterial and pull impurities from the skin. For example, if you are stung by a bee or bitten by an insect you can cut an onion in half and hold it on the wound for about 10 minutes. You'll want to do this as soon as possible to get as much of the toxins out as you can. Onions have many other properties as well. They can be used to aid digestion, help prevent hardening of the arteries, treat sore throats, bronchitis and asthma, among other things. They are a useful food and medicine to have around. Onions have even shown benefits in treating some forms of cancer.

Parsley ~ Parsley, like the members of the Mint family, is naturally astringent. It can also be soothing and healing for those who suffer with bad cases of acne, eczema and psoriasis. Ever wonder why restaurants put Parsley as a garnish on the plates? It's not just there to look pretty. Parsley freshens your breath after a meal. Parsley also makes a good rinse for all hair types.

Plantain ~ This common yard "weed" is actually very useful. It can be used in creams or salves to help heal minor scrapes and cuts. I have used it directly on the skin to help stop the bleeding of a wound. Plantain is abundant everywhere. It can be found all around urban areas. It is rich in Vitamin A, C, and K as well as Magnesium.

According to GreenMedInfo.com "Studies have shown that plantain has anti-inflammatory effects, and it is also rich in tannins (which helps draw tissues together to stop bleeding) and allantoin (a compound that promotes healing of injured skin cells). Further studies have indicated that plantain may also reduce blood pressure, and that the seeds of the plant may reduce blood cholesterol levels. Plantain seeds were also widely used as a natural laxative, given their high source of fiber. Teas made from the plant, were used to treat diarrhea, dysentery, intestinal worms, and bleeding mucous membranes. The roots were also recommended for relieving toothaches and headaches as well as healing poor gums."

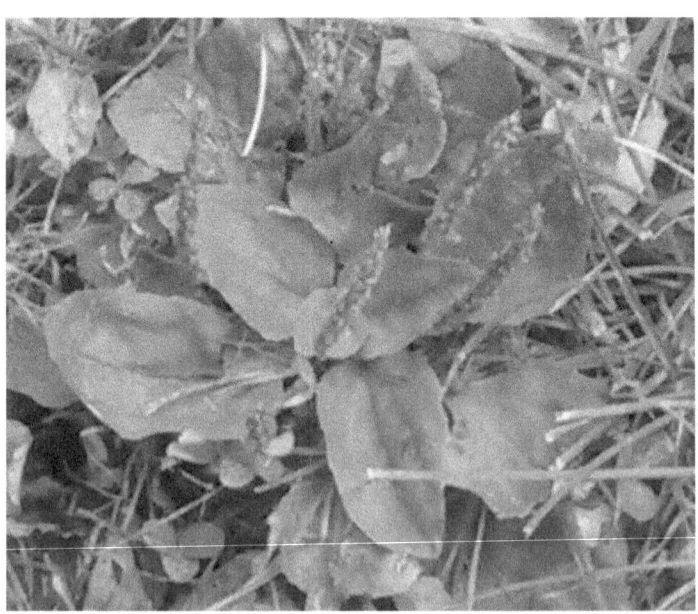

Peppermint ~ Peppermint is invigorating, cooling, anti-inflammatory, analgesic and mildly antiseptic. It's good for helping to get rid of aches and pains as well as controlling bacteria on the skin.

Raspberry ~ Raspberry leaf tea has been used to help many women's issues. It is said to help with hormone imbalances, menstrual cramps as well as childbirth. You can find it often combined with Nettle.

Rose ~ Roses have long been associated with love and beauty. The essence of Roses has been used for centuries for such things as relieving Depression and grief, attracting love and passion, as an aphrodisiac as well as symbolizing beauty. Some say that Rose oil is one of the first essential oils documented for use. You can use them to make Rose water which can be a wonderful toner to the skin, especially when combined with glycerine. If you decide that you would like to try to make your own Rose water make sure to use organically grown Roses so that you won't be adding pesticides and other harsh chemicals to your skin.

Rosemary ~ Rosemary has astringent, antiseptic, anti-inflammatory, nervine, carminative, diuretic, antidepressant, circulatory stimulant, antispasmodic, detoxifying and stimulating properties. It helps to rid the skin of impurities by opening the pores and helps to prevent wrinkles. It is very helpful for oily skin and is a strong antioxidant. Rosemary is known to improve circulation as well as promoting hair growth, conditioning hair and preventing dandruff. It is a good herb to use in sore or sprained muscle rubs.

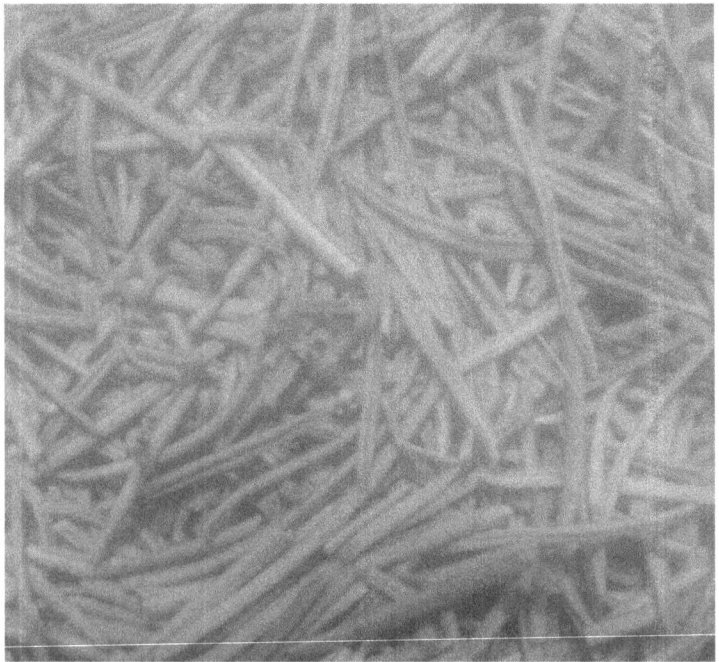

Dried Rosemary leaves from my spice cabinet.

Sage ~ Sage has been used to darken and tone hair as well as being a hair growth stimulant. It also has antibacterial properties. Sage has been used for its carminative (anti-gas) properties as well as to relieve stomach pain, diarrhea, bloating, heartburn, Depression and memory loss. It can be used to slow milk production in mothers and to reduce hot flashes caused by menopause.

Tea Tree – Tea Tree Oil is also known as Melaleuca oil and is native to Australia. It is my second favorite oil, next to Lavender. It is antiseptic, antifungal, antibacterial and antiviral. It is easily absorbed by the skin and, along with Lavender, can be used neat (by itself, without diluting in a carrier oil). I use a few drops of it in shampoo to help with dandruff. Tea Tree has been used as an antiseptic, fungicide and germicide.

Thyme ~ Thyme is antifungal, antiseptic, anti-inflammatory, anti-parasitic, expectorant, an immune booster and also is a lung cleanser. Because of its expectorant and lung cleansing properties it is often used for whooping cough, bronchitis, asthma and other ailments related to breathing and/or congestion. It used

95

to be given, in tea form, to women who had just given birth in order to expel the placenta. It can also be made into a paste by mashing up the fresh leaves, or dried leaves combined with water or other liquid, and applied as a poultice.

Turmeric ~ This is a spice that should be easy to find in your local grocery store. It is often used to prevent wrinkles due to its anti-allergic, antiseptic, antioxidant and nerve and blood vessel stimulating properties.

Valerian ~ The root of the Valerian plant is the most commonly used. It is touted as a nervine and a sedative. It can be used for someone who suffers from anxiety issues or to help you get to sleep at night. It helps to reduce stress, nervous tension, Depression, irritability, hysteria, panic, anxiety, fear, stomach cramping, indigestion due to nervousness, delusions, exhaustion, and, of course, nervous sleeplessness. It is even said to help in cases of sciatica, multiple sclerosis, epilepsy, shingles, and peripheral neuropathy, including numbness, tingling, muscle weakness, and pain in the extremities. It has been said that it can even help with behavioral problems in both adults and children, and is

96

used to treat attention deficit disorders, hyperactivity and anxiety headaches. I have used it myself to help treat a child with Attention Deficit Hyperactivity Disorder (ADHD).

Witch Hazel ~ Many of you may be familiar with Witch Hazel already but did you know it has toning, astringent, antiseptic and anti-inflammatory properties? It is soothing to irritated skin and doesn't dry it out. It also helps to prevent wrinkles by toning and refreshing the skin. It is much better to use on oily skin than alcohol which dries the skin out and can cause it to produce even more oil.

Yarrow ~ Yarrow is astringent and anti-inflammatory. It is used often with acne prone skin. It can also be used as a sitz bath for those suffering from hemorrhoids. It can be used on wounds to help stop bleeding. I like to make a salve with it, combined with Plantain, to help with minor cuts, scrapes and bruises.

How to make Infusions and Decoctions by Starr Morgayne

Products You Can Purchase

You can purchase these products and more by checking out https://www.etsy.com/shop/NaturalSelectionWB

None of these items have been evaluated by the FDA and are not intended to diagnose, cure, or treat any ailment or illness. We also take requests for custom blends.

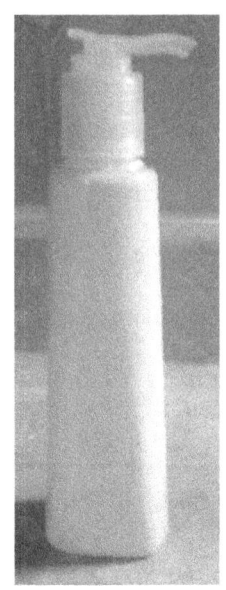

Sole Soothing Foot Lotion $10 + S&H
8 oz bottle with pump top (shape and color may vary)

This lotion feels great and works even better. Being a Diabetic I was looking for something that would soften the rough skin on my heels. After searching and searching I finally decided to take matters into my own hands. I created this lotion and have never looked back. It contains Aloe Vera, Cocoa Butter and Calendula Petals to soften and heal the skin. It also contains Comfrey leaves for their skin rejuvenating properties. I've also added Tea Tree and Lavender Oils for their antifungal, antiseptic and antibiotic attributes along with Peppermint Oil for its cooling and circulatory benefits.
Ingredients: Aloe Vera Juice, Cocoa Butter, Vegetable glycerine, Olive Oil, Emulsifying Wax, Calendula Petals, Comfrey Leaves, Lavender Buds, Lavender Essential Oil, Tea Tree Essential Oil, Peppermint Essential Oil

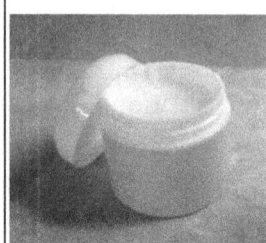

ACE Face and Eye Cream $5 + S&H
2 oz walled jar with lid (color may vary)

This natural skin cream is perfect for revitalizing maturing skin or maintaining younger looking skin. It contains vitamins A, C, and E mixed in Coconut Oil to enhance the elasticity in your skin. It repairs skin tissue and damage. It softens skin, moisturizes, and reduces the appearance of scarring, wrinkles, and stretch marks. I have had some great reviews on its benefits for those with Rosacea also!

Ingredients: Organic extra virgin Coconut Oil, glycerine, water, Vitamin E, Vitamin C, Vitamin A

All Natural Antibiotic First Aid Ointment $3 + S&H
¼ oz container with lid

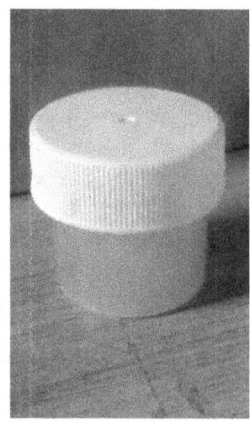

This is a first aid ointment or salve that can be used for cuts, scrapes, bruises, abrasions, etc. It was made using all natural ingredients.

The herbs used in this product are used for these purposes:
• Tea Tree Oil: antibiotic, anti-fungal, antiviral, antibacterial
• Lavender: analgesic (pain relief), antibiotic, anti-fungal, antiviral, antibacterial
• Lemon: antibiotic, antifungal, antiviral, antibacterial
Ingredients: Extra Virgin Olive Oil, Beeswax, Vitamin E, Lavender Essential Oil, Tea Tree Essential Oil, Lemon Essential Oil, Calendula Petals, Comfrey Leaf

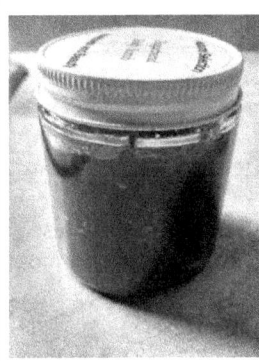

Gingerbread Body Scrub $5 + S&H
4 oz glass jar with lid

This is an all natural body scrub that smells heavenly. Perfect for a gift for yourself or someone you love. Extra Virgin Olive Oil is a great moisturizer for the skin. Sugar is an excellent exfoliant and the spices used in this scrub can help with circulation. As with all products, some settling may occur. Just stir and use.

Ingredients: Brown Sugar, Cinnamon, Nutmeg, Ginger, Cloves, essential oils, Extra Virgin Olive Oil, Sugar

Pumpkin Pie Body Scrub $5 + S&H
4 oz walled jar with lid

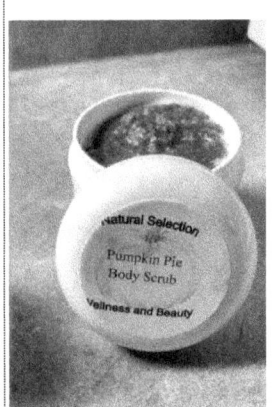

This is an all natural body scrub that smells heavenly. Perfect for a gift for yourself or someone you love. Coconut Oil and Honey are great moisturizers for the skin. Sugar is an excellent exfoliant and the spices used in this scrub can help with circulation. As with all products, some settling may occur. Just stir and use. Due to the fact that this body scrub contains Coconut Oil it will solidify at lower temperatures.

Ingredients: Coconut Oil, brown Sugar, Honey, pumpkin pie spices, Cinnamon, Nutmeg, Ginger

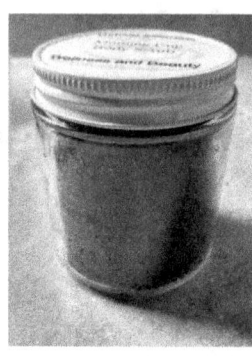

Morning Cup Body Scrub $5 + S&H
4 oz glass jar with lid

This is a wonderful body scrub that will invigorate you! The coffee and the Peppermint in this scrub will wake you right up. The caffeine in the coffee grounds has also been shown to reduce the appearance and formation of cellulite so there's an added bonus! Great for every morning, especially those mornings when you just can't seem to rise and shine.

Ingredients: Coffee beans, Olive Oil, Peppermint Essential Oil, Salt

Cleansing Grains Face Scrub $4 + S&H
2 oz glass jar with lid

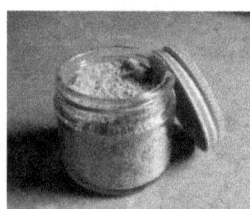

This facial scrub is gentle on sensitive facial skin but great for exfoliating. Combine a little with water or whole milk and scrub gently to reduce redness, oil, puffiness and signs of aging.

Ingredients: Oats, Almonds, Rose petals, Lavender, Kaolin clay

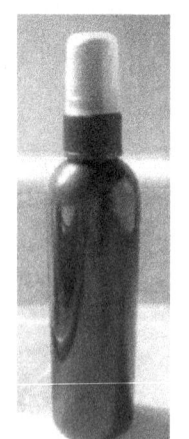

Soothing Burn Spray $8 + S&H
4 oz spray bottle

This is an excellent spray for any type of burn. If stored in the refrigerator it adds a refreshing coolness to the spray. Excellent for spraying on sunburns or other minor burns or wounds.

Bottle color may vary.

Ingredients: Aloe Vera Juice, Lavender Essential Oil, Vitamin E

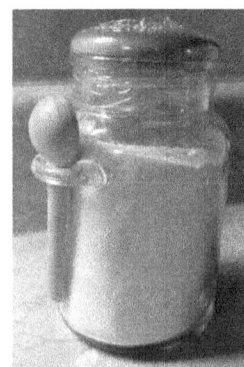

Lavender Milk Bath $10 + S&H
Wooden corked bottle with spoon

Milk is a soothing, moisturizing, yet non-greasy bath additive that gently soothes and cleanses your child's skin. A warm Lavender aromatherapy bath does wonders for a fussy baby or toddler (or even Mommy). Comes in a gorgeous glass jar with a wooden lid and wooden spoon attached on the side.

To use: Use the little wooden spoon to sprinkle a small amount in a warm bath

Ingredients: Lavender, milk, cornstarch

Companies

Natural Selection Wellness and Beauty
P.O. Box 11496
Fort Wayne, Indiana 46858-1496
USA
https://www.etsy.com/people/naturalselectionwb
NaturalSelectionWB@gmail.com

THAYERS Natural Remedies
P.O. Box 56
Westport, Connecticut 06881-0056
USA
http://www.thayers.com

Mountain Rose Herbs
P.O. Box 50220
Eugene, OR 97405
USA
http://www.mountainroseherbs.com

Frontier Natural Foods Co-op
P.O. Box 299
3021 78th St.
Norway, IA 52318
USA
http://www.frontiercoop.com/

How to make Infusions and Decoctions by Starr Morgayne

Index

119

Suggested Reading

Here are several books that I would recommend for doing some research on your own. This is by no means an extensive list.

Buhner, Stephen Harrod, *Herbal Antibiotics; Natural Alternatives for Treating Drug-Resistant Bacteria*, Storey Books, 1999

Foster, Steven, *101 Medicinal Herbs; An Illustrated Guide*, Interweave Press, 1998

Gladstar, Rosemary, *Herbal Healing for Women; Simple Home Remedies for Women of All Ages*, Simon & Schuster, 1993

Keville, Kathi, *Herbs for Health and Healing*, Rodale Press, Inc., 1996

Kowalchik, Claire and Hylton, William H. (editors), *Rodale's Illustrated Encyclopedia of Herbs*, Rodale Press, 1987

Mars, Brigitte, Herbalist AHG, *Dandelion Medicine; Remedies and Recipes to Detoxify, Nourish, Stimulate*, Storey Books, 1999

Morgayne, Starr, *Bewitching Beauty; Bringing out your inner Goddess, naturally*, Dark Moon Press, 2010

Murray, Michael N.D. and Pizzorno, Joseph N.D., *Encyclopedia of Natural Medicine*, Revised 2nd Edition, Prima Publishing, 1998

Rose, Jeanne, *Herbs & Aromatherapy for the Reproductive System*, Frog Ltd., 1994

Royal, Penny C., *Herbally Yours*, Third Edition, Sound Nutrition, 1982

Smyth, Angela, *The Complete Home Healer; Your Guide to Every Treatment Available for over 300 of the Most Common Health Problems*, HarperCollins Publishers, 1994

Telesco, Patricia, *The Herbal Arts; A Handbook of Gardening, Recipes, Healing, Crafts, and Spirituality*, Carol Publishing Group, 1998

Trattler, Dr. Ross, N.D., D.O., *Better Health through Natural Healing; How To Get Well Without Drugs or Surgery*, Second Edition, Hinkler Books Pty Ltd, 2001

Walker, Dr. Lynne Paige and Brown, Ellen Hodgson J.D., *Nature's Pharmacy; Break the Drug Cycle with Safe Natural Treatments for 200 Everyday Ailments*, Reward Books, 1998

Weed, Susun S, *Wise Woman Herbal for the Childbearing Year*, Ash Tree Publishing, 1986

White, Linda B., M.D. and Mavor, Sunny A.H.G, *Kids, Herbs, Health*, Interweave Press, 1998

How to make Infusions and Decoctions by Starr Morgayne

About the Author

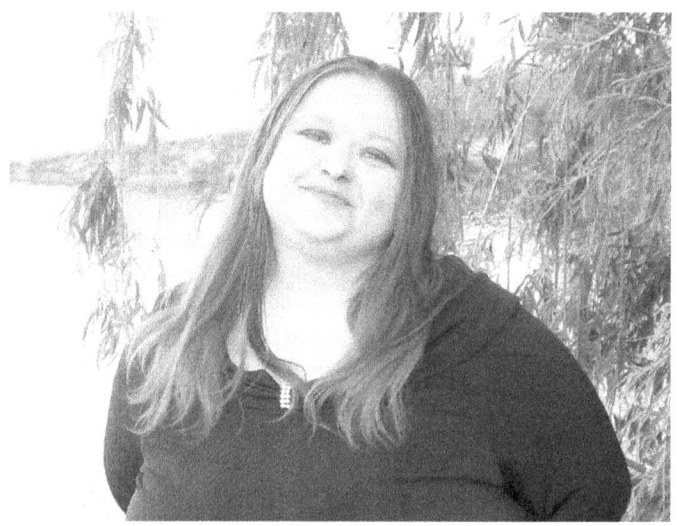

Starr Morgayne is in her thirties and has been studying herbs and alternative healing methods for more than 15 years. She is a Certified Herbalist and is working to obtain a degree in Naturopathy.

She lives in Indiana with her four cats, three dogs, two ferrets, lots of fish and her loving family.

In her spare time she enjoys writing, reading, photography, crafting and gardening.

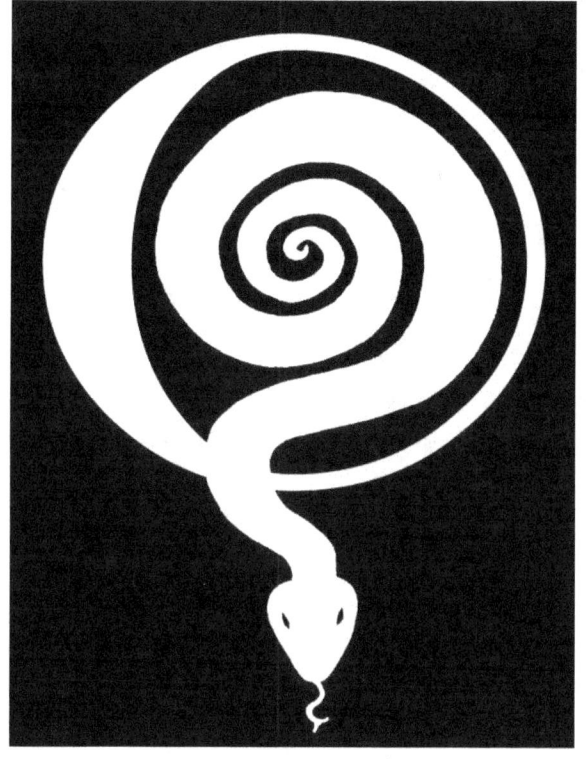

Dark Moon Press

P.O. Box 11496

Fort Wayne, Indiana 46858-1496

DarkMoon@darkmoonpress.com

www.darkmoonpress.com

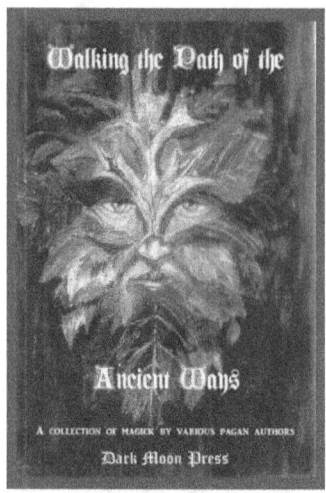

Walking the Path of the Ancient Ways; a collection of magic by various pagan authors
Corvis Nocturnum

Pagan authors from various backgrounds share their story on being pagan in the modern world. Insightful and thought provoking. With writings by Starr Morgayne, Corvis Nocturnum, Andrieh Vitimus and many more known and new voices.
ISBN-13: 978-1470034641

200 pages
9.99 USD

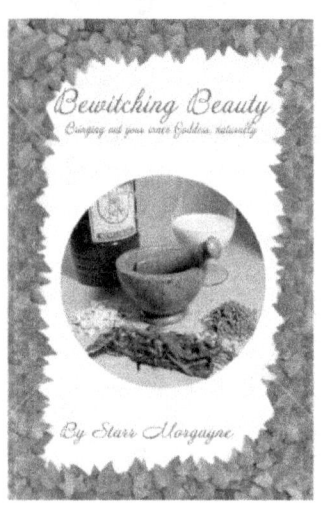

addition to your journey.

Bewitching Beauty: Bringing out your inner Goddess, naturally
Starr Morgayne

Women of all ages are concerned about their skin, their bodies and growing older. In this book the author offers simple yet effective, personally tested recipes based on readily available ingredients, and her own unique perspective to help get you in touch with Mother Nature and yourself. Regardless of what stage of life you are in this book can be a positive

ISBN-13: 978-1451585872
200 pages
$16.95 USD

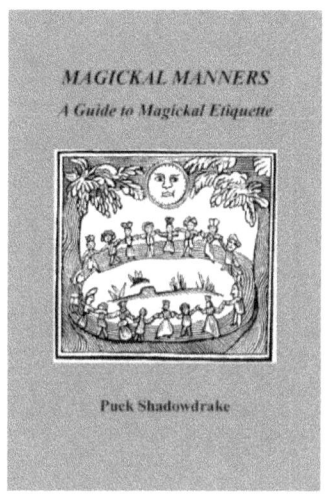

MAGICKAL MANNERS: A Guide to Magickal Etiquette
Puck Shadowdrake

"An extensive overview of the practices and etiquette of the entire Neo Pagan community. An excellent resource for chaplains as well as for students seeking a spiritual path." Kerr Cuhulain, author of *Pagan Religions: A Handbook for Diversity Training*
ISBN-13: 978-1481910958
600 pages
$39.99 USD

JOURNEYS FROM THE MEADOW: A Book of Guided Mediations
Puck Shadowdrake

Puck Shadowdrake, the author of *MAGICKAL MANNERS: A Guide to Magickal Etiquette* brings you his collection of meditations to guide the modern witch through their various journeys through the path for relaxation, healing the body and contacting your deities, spirit guides and much more.
Pages: TBA
Price: $19.99 USD
Spring 2014

www.ingramcontent.com/pod-product-compliance
Lightning Source LLC
Chambersburg PA
CBHW070920290526

45795CB00001B/366